Craniosacral Chi Kung

Craniosacral Chi Kung

Integrating Body and Emotion in the Cosmic Flow

Mantak Chia
and Joyce Thom

Destiny Books
Rochester, Vermont • Toronto, Canada

Destiny Books
One Park Street
Rochester, Vermont 05767
www.DestinyBooks.com

Destiny Books is a division of Inner Traditions International

Originally published in Thailand in 2014 by Universal Tao Publications under the title *CranioSacral Chi Kung: Connecting with the Cosmic Flow*

Library of Congress Cataloging-in-Publication Data
Names: Chia, Mantak, 1944- | Thom, Joyce.
Title: Craniosacral chi kung : integrating body and emotion in the cosmic flow / Mantak Chia and Joyce Thom.
Description: Rochester, Vermont : Destiny Books, [2016] | "Originally published in Thailand in 2014 by Universal Tao Publications under the title CranioSacral Chi Kung: connecting with the cosmic flow"—Title page verso. | Includes bibliographical references and index.
Identifiers: LCCN 2015016319| ISBN 9781620554234 (paperback) | ISBN 9781620554241 (ebook)
Subjects: LCSH: Craniosacral therapy. | Qi gong. | Mind and body. | BISAC: HEALTH & FITNESS / Massage & Reflexotherapy. | HEALTH & FITNESS / Acupressure & Acupuncture (see also MEDICAL / Acupuncture). | BODY, MIND & SPIRIT / Healing / Energy (Chi Kung, Reiki, Polarity).
Classification: LCC RZ399.C73 C45 2016 | DDC 615.8/3—dc23

Printed and bound in the United States by Versa Press, Inc.

10 9 8 7 6 5 4 3 2

Text design by Priscilla Baker and layout by Debbie Glogover
This book was typeset in Garamond Premier Pro with Present and Futura Std used as display typefaces

Illustrations by Udon Jandee
Photographs by Sopitnapa Promnon

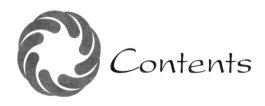

Contents

Acknowledgments   xi

Putting Craniosacral Chi Kung into Practice   xiii

Introduction   1

PART ONE
Physical Flow

1 • Working with Cosmic Flow: Western and Taoist
  Approaches   9

2 • Awakening the Major Pumps   25

3 • Building Awareness and Appreciation   64

PART TWO
Emotional and Mental Flows

4 • Everything Is Connected to the Flow   81

5 • Balancing Emotional and Mental Flows   99

PART THREE

Spiritual Flow

6 • Everything Is Energy   142

7 • Becoming Liquid Light: The Endocrine System and
      Spiritual Practice   191

8 • Cosmic Flow: The Art and Skill of Nondoing   224

Appendix 1. Cosmic Cranial-Elemental Connections   240

Appendix 2. Additional Pumps   248

Notes   250

Bibliography   252

Online Resources   256

About the Authors   259

The Universal Healing Tao System
and Training Center   262

Index   264

List of Practices Covered in Craniosacral Chi Kung

- **Chapter 2 – Awakening the Major Pumps**

  Natural or Abdominal Breathing   28

  Reverse Breathing   29

  Tapping into the Heart   34

  Chi Kung Breath of Life   37

  Breathing into the Heart   39

  Opening the Waist   48

  Opening the Hips   48

  Rotating the Sacrum   49

  Awakening the Sacral Pump   50

  Filling the Sacral Pump   52

  Rocking the Neck   54

  Bending the Neck   54

  Rotating the Neck   55

  Rolling the Neck   56

  Activating the Cranial Pump   56

  Spinal Cord Breathing   58

  Crane   60

  Turtle   61

  Wagging the Dragon's Tail   62

- **Chapter 3 – Building Awareness and Appreciation**

  Following the Breath   64

  Listening to the Heart Flow   66

  Connecting to the Core Link   68

  Connecting the Pumps   72

Appreciating the Pumps   *76*

Sustaining the Flow   *77*

● **Chapter 5 – Balancing Emotional and Mental Flows**

Push Hands: Listening   *105*

Push Hands: Following   *107*

Push Hands: Noticing the Direction of Movement   *108*

Push Hands: Unwinding   *109*

Yin Breathing   *115*

Listening with the Heart to Your Psoas Muscle   *116*

Psoas Muscle Release   *118*

Empty Force Breathing   *122*

Unwinding the Flow Using Chi Nei Tsang Self-Massage   *124*

Laughter Chi Kung   *128*

Metal Element: The Lungs' Sound   *130*

Water Element: The Kidneys' Sound   *132*

Wood Element: The Liver's Sound   *133*

Fire Element: The Heart's Sound   *135*

Earth Element: The Spleen's Sound   *136*

The Triple Warmer's Sound   *138*

● **Chapter 6 – Everything Is Energy**

Shaking the Bones   *146*

Feeling Cranial Motility   *152*

Following the Clock   *161*

Bone Breathing   *169*

Cranial Bone Sensing   *170*

Riding the Horse   *172*

Swimming Dragon   *173*

Fire Dragon   *174*

Microcosmic Orbit   175

Brushing the Yin and Yang Meridians   180

Tracing the Meridian Flow   182

● **Chapter 7 – Becoming Liquid Light**

Warm-Ups for the World Link Meditation:
  Sensing the Cranial Wave   214

Combining the Three Tan Tiens:
  Moving into Fluid Tide   215

Expanding to the Six Directions:
  Connecting to the Long Tide   216

● **Chapter 8 – Cosmic Flow**

Yin and Yang Breathing   225

Flowing between Empty and Full   228

Push Hands: Moving Into Stillness   231

Pull the Bow and Shoot the Arrow   234

Becoming the Cosmic Flow   237

● **Appendix 1 – Cosmic Cranial-Elemental Connections**

Cosmic Cranial-Elemental Meditation   241

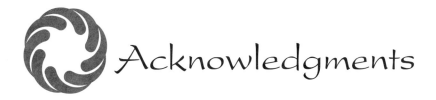

Acknowledgments

The authors would like to express our gratitude to the many Taoist masters who have generously and patiently shared their wisdom, experience, and practices over the generations. Their devotion to the Taoist arts and commitment to the unbroken oral transmission of this special lineage of Taoist knowledge has made this book possible. In particular, Master Chia would like to thank Yi Eng for his abundant teachings, which had such a deep influence on the development of the Universal Healing Tao practices.

Additionally, we would like to thank the many teachers and practitioners from the osteopathic, craniosacral, and Chinese medicine lineages for their contributions to those arts and the writing of this book. Joyce is particularly grateful to Hugh Milne, Brian O'Dea, and Ou Yang Min for deepening her learning and growth in these areas. She would also like to acknowledge Steve Schumacher for his valuable insights and feedback and Ching Fung Dao Shr for his profound teachings.

We are also grateful for our families, friends, and communities for their warm support as well as for their inspiration and encouragement.

We thank the many contributors essential to this book's final form: the editorial and production staff at Inner Traditions/Destiny Books for their efforts to clarify the text and produce this handsome new edition of the book, and Gail Rex for her line edit of the new edition.

We wish to thank Colin Drown for his assistance in producing the earlier editions of this book, particularly for his superb editorial work and invaluable assistance with the graphics and illustrations.

And special thanks to our Thai production team: Hirunyathorn Punsan, Sopitnapa Promnon, and Udon Jandee.

Putting Craniosacral Chi Kung into Practice

The information presented in this book is based on the authors' personal experience and knowledge of Inner Alchemy practices. The practices described in this book have been used successfully for thousands of years by Taoists trained by personal instruction. Readers should not undertake the practices without receiving personal transmission and training from a certified instructor of the Universal Healing Tao, since certain of these practices, if done improperly, may cause injury or result in health problems. This book is intended to supplement individual training by the Universal Healing Tao and to serve as a reference guide for these practices. Anyone who undertakes these practices on the basis of this book alone does so entirely at his or her own risk.

The meditations, practices, and techniques described herein are not intended to be used as an alternative or substitute for professional medical treatment and care. If any readers are suffering from illnesses based on mental or emotional disorders, an appropriate professional health care practitioner or therapist should be consulted. Such problems should be corrected before you start Universal Healing Tao training.

Neither the Universal Healing Tao nor its staff and instructors can be responsible for the consequences of any practice or misuse of the information contained in this book. If the reader undertakes any exercise without strictly following the instructions, notes, and warnings, the responsibility must lie solely with the reader.

This book does not attempt to give any medical diagnosis, treatment, prescription, or remedial recommendation in relation to any human disease, ailment, suffering, or physical condition whatsoever.

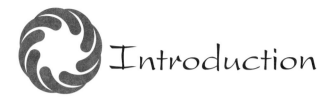 # Introduction

One winter, Joyce was at Tao Garden for a series of Universal Healing Tao retreats. Throughout the weeks of intensive Taoist practices, Master Chia frequently emphasized the importance of the cranial and sacral pumps. As a practitioner of both Craniosacral Work and Chi Kung, Joyce was deeply interested in the resonance between these two practices, and how well they complemented each other in providing a deep understanding of the foundations of health and well-being. Fascinated by modern support for the ancient practices he has devoted his life to sharing, Master Chia felt that a book about the overlap and common principles between these Eastern and Western practices would be immensely valuable to a wide audience. That book is the one you are now reading.

CHI KUNG AND CRANIOSACRAL WORK
A Common Approach

On the surface, it may seem as if there is little in common between modern science and the ancient wisdom traditions. Yet, rather than opposing each other, scientific research and new technology offer opportunities for us to enhance our understanding and appreciation of the ancient ways.

At the root of both Taoism and Craniosacral Work is a focus on cultivating harmonious, balanced movement on all levels. A core belief of both systems is that healthy internal movement automatically translates into greater harmony between the individual and his or her external environment. Based on this shared perspective, both practices emphasize a concept we refer to here as *Flow:* the natural, effortless unfolding of our lives in a way that moves us toward wholeness and harmony.

Flow is central to both Taoism and Craniosacral Work because it is essential to our health and well-being. Communication and coordination between all of our parts require the smooth flow of biochemical and electromagnetic signals through our fluids, tissues, and bones. The fluidity of our emotions and thoughts enables us to harmonize our inner world and to be flexible and resilient in our dealings with the outer world. The movement of chi is what moves us through life.

Both cosmologies believe that optimal Flow is synonymous with

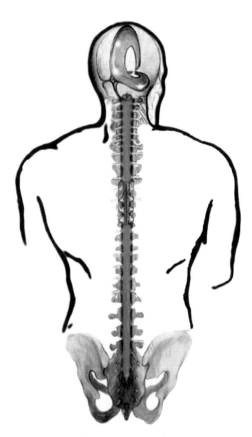

Fig. I.1. The craniosacral connection

health and harmony, and that each person has an inherent capacity to heal—to return to the natural state of optimal Flow. Each system offers simple techniques to increase awareness of that Flow and powerful practices for balancing and enhancing it. This book draws on Taoist and Western lineages—both ancient and modern—to explore the nature of Flow and practices for improving it.

HOW TO USE THIS BOOK

The following pages offer easy and practical exercises for finding, generating, and sustaining Flow on many levels. The book provides clear and detailed guidance for beginning practitioners, as well as a wealth of new information to deepen the understanding and experience of advanced practitioners.

No prior knowledge of Chi Kung, Craniosacral Work, bodywork, or anatomy is required to understand this book. Some readers will get the most out of it by reading it cover to cover in order to understand the theory, anatomy, and exercises. Others will want to focus first on experiencing greater Flow through the powerful exercises, and will return later to deepen their contextual understanding once they have felt the firsthand effects of their practice. To make it easier to find the exercises and for later reference, we have included a list of practices immediately following the table of contents.

The book will guide you in:

- Understanding each of the different pumping systems and easily balancing the flow through each system
- Experiencing the flow inherent in Taoist Chi Kung practices
- Tapping effortlessly into the power of the lesser and greater flows and benefitting from better physical, emotional, mental, energetic, and spiritual flow
- Connecting deeply with the transcendent primordial Flow

The first three chapters set the context and establish the foundation for awakening, becoming aware of, and appreciating Flow in our lives. You will learn how to activate the major pumps and how to generate and sustain their flows. Chapters 4 and 5 discuss ways of harmonizing and enhancing your internal physical, emotional, and mental flows.

In chapter 6, you'll move deeper into Flow by looking at the movement and energy of your bones, which are doorways to deeper ancestral and lineage flows. You'll learn to sense your bones and breathe with them to access the wisdom they offer. You will practice unifying your individual energy fields and augmenting the internal flow of chi with Microcosmic Orbit and meridian meditations.

After enhancing the flows within and building your energetic foundation, you'll turn your attention to connecting with even larger flows in chapter 7. The discussion of waves and tides offers a craniosacral

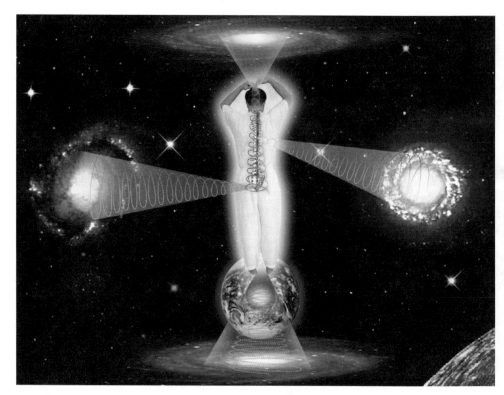

Fig. I.2. Cosmic chi flow

perspective on how Chi Kung practices provide a methodical way to change our level of consciousness and develop our spirituality. The exercises at the end of the chapter will help you integrate your new understanding of both the mechanics and the magic of spiritual flow. The final chapter invites you to explore the balance of yang and yin in doing and not doing. When you become one with the cosmic Flow, you return effortlessly to your primordial state of wholeness, health, and Oneness.

Craniosacral Chi Kung provides Chi Kung practitioners and spiritual seekers with a scientific physiological context for why Chi Kung and meditation are so effective. For bodyworkers, these practices offer a critical self-care component that is often missing from their training. The exercises will not only deepen their understanding of their own bodies and improve their own health, but also provide useful self-care homework for their clients. More than just conceptual information, *Craniosacral Chi Kung* offers insights and practical exercises for finding, generating, and sustaining Flow in our daily lives.

PART ONE

Physical Flow

Part 1 introduces the concepts of Flow from the Taoist and Western craniosacral perspectives. The individual chapters explore the importance of Flow to our physical, emotional, and mental health. They also explain the assessment of Flow as understood in the craniosacral approach, which considers tempo, magnitude, balance, and quality.

After learning to assess Flow, we will explore the four major pumps that activate it: the cardiac, respiratory, cranial, and sacral pumping systems that circulate fluids, nutrients, and energies throughout the body. We will build awareness of these pumps through our kinesthetic sense of the connection and flow among them. For some of us, the craniosacral connection has been disrupted by injury, illness, or lifestyle issues. As you practice moving the cranium and sacrum together in a harmonious, synchronous way, you will build new neural network communication pathways (or strengthen existing ones), which will help you become more fluid and integrated on multiple levels. As a result, you will not only move differently but also feel more connected with your body in deeper and more profound ways.

In addition to physical exercises, we'll also use guided meditations to experience Flow in our bones, tissues, and fluids, and to enhance our awareness of those flows. In so doing, we increase our ability to track and adjust these flows as needed. For example, if you become aware that you are tired and your throat is sore, you can rest and take Vitamin C so that you do not get sick. Likewise, if you notice less flow at certain times or in particular areas, you can meditate or do your practices to cultivate and generate more chi and greater flow, increasing your resilience and vitality.

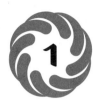

Working with Cosmic Flow

Western and Taoist Approaches

The dictionary definition of *flow* is "to move in a steady and continuous way; to circulate; to proceed smoothly and readily."[1] In a larger context, we might say that while we are "in the flow," we are focused, engaged, and energized, and that our actions feel purposeful, enjoyable, and effortless. If you think of a time when you felt "in the zone"—perhaps playing sports, creating something, having an "on" day of great efficiency at work, playing music, or practicing Chi Kung—and remember how that felt, you can connect with the feeling of Flow.

Intuitively, we understand that being "in the flow" is beneficial, but getting there can be challenging. Flow can be present—or absent—on physical, emotional, mental, energetic, and spiritual levels. While Western medicine acknowledges the link between good health and good circulation through the body's pumping systems, it does not suggest many ways to improve those flows other than exercise.

TAOIST COSMIC FLOW

Because energy flow is an essential element of Taoism, Chi Kung practices have focused for thousands of years on improving it. Taoism's

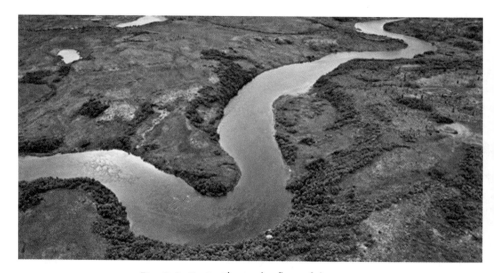

Fig. 1.1. Taoist Flow—the flow of the river

emphasis on harmonious flow is relevant in today's world, not only for our health, but also for our relationships, careers, and personal growth. By using Chi Kung to balance flow, we can become more healthy, connected, abundant, and energized.

CRANIOSACRAL FLOW

Craniosacral Work is a Western holistic healing modality, based on osteopathy, that optimizes the flow of energy throughout the body. The name refers to practitioners' attention to the craniosacral rhythm, which is the flow of cerebrospinal fluid from the head (cranium) to the tailbone (sacrum). This rhythmic movement is generated by pressure changes throughout the head and spine during the production and absorption of cerebrospinal fluid; its subtle flow indicates the harmony or disharmony of the whole person (fig. 1.2).

By working with the body's inherent healing processes to restore the natural movement of the fluids, tissues, and bones, craniosacral practitioners can assist their clients to release painful or restricted conditions anywhere in the system. By bringing greater awareness to the internal

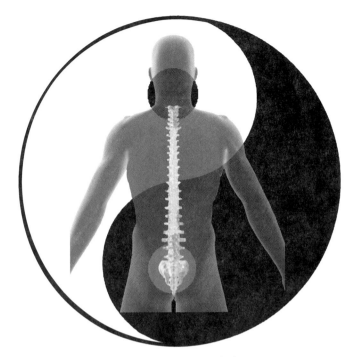

Fig. 1.2. Craniosacral Flow

flows of the client, craniosacral practitioners facilitate and empower the client's self-healing process. Craniosacral Work can be helpful in calming the mind, harmonizing the emotions, and encouraging physical well-being. Like Chi Kung practices, the meditative states that occur with Craniosacral Work facilitate a deeper mind-body-spirit connection that is healing and deeply rejuvenating on all levels.

THE PHYSICAL BENEFITS OF FLOW

On a basic physical level, Flow is critically important for providing the connection, communication, and resilience that our systems need to function.

Connection: In order to live, we need to keep oxygen, blood, and nutrients moving through our bodies. Movement bathes each of the body's structures, bringing nourishment to organs, tissues, and bones. Like a highway system with open roads and flowing traffic, a well-connected body allows vital supplies to move from where they are produced to where they are needed. On an energy level, Flow connects and distributes vital chi to all parts of body.

Communication: Using another analogy, the Internet, we can see how Flow allows information to be shared effortlessly. Healthy flow enables one part of the body to communicate with other parts so that coordination, action, and good decision-making can take place. Without the flow of information through the sensory nervous system, for example, we wouldn't notice sensations critical for our health like pain or pleasure, hunger or satiation, hot or cold. The brain then uses this information to make decisions and take action: communication along our motor nerves tells our muscles to move.

Resilience: Resilience is the ability to be strong, healthy, and successful when encountering challenges. When our energies are flowing appropriately, our systems can adjust dynamically to changes and optimize themselves. When water meets an obstacle, it adjusts "fluidly"—perhaps by going around, moving through, sinking below, or eventually eroding the obstacle. Water is only unable to continue on its path when there is insufficient flow. The practices of Taoism and Craniosacral Work cultivate the inherent wisdom of the body and its propensity to return toward health whenever possible. Flow facilitates this intelligent process of adaptation and ongoing rebalancing.

Flow and Our Health

In the West, science uses machines, such as the electrocardiogram (ECG) and electroencephalogram (EEG), to measure the rhythms and flows of the body's shifting electromagnetic field. Through research and study, medicine has established the average ranges for healthy individuals and uses readings outside those ranges to flag potential health issues.

Much of Taoist practice is based on the notion that chi or life-force energy must flow to be healthy. If energy becomes stagnant, blocked, or weakened, our health is adversely affected. Traditionally, Asian physicians assess the movement of chi in the meridians, tissues, organs, and bones by feeling the pulses. By listening to the quality of these flows, a skilled practitioner would know what issues were arising and how to be of assistance in helping to resolve them. In this cosmology, pain and disease are believed to result directly from poor flow—movement that is either excessive or deficient. Conversely, health and harmony come from abundant chi that is flowing in a balanced way through all the systems.

THE BROADER BENEFITS OF FLOW

From the simple pulsations of single-celled amoebas to the multi-year migrations of the whales, life on this planet is organized around rhythms and flows. In humans, our internal pumping systems circulate oxygen, blood, and cerebrospinal fluid throughout the body.

On a larger scale, the planets rotate and move in their orbits, the seasons flow from one to another, the tides ebb and swell with the waxing and waning of the moon, and day flows into night and back again (fig. 1.3). Because we are connected with heaven and earth, each of

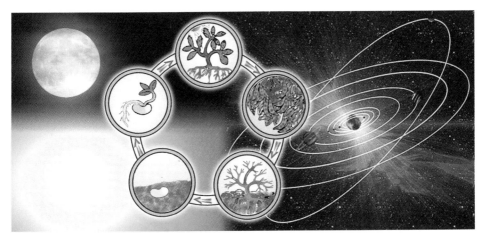

Fig. 1.3. Natural flows

these rhythms affects our own flows: we are attuned to these cycles, following them in ways we may not even be aware of. For example, science has long acknowledged that circadian rhythms influence our sleep and feeding patterns. And we intuitively notice that we are more active in the spring than we are in the winter.

When we are in the Flow, we are in tune with these larger rhythms; things seem to unfold synchronistically and effortlessly for us. Being in the Flow brings us to places of exhilaration, accelerated growth, and enhanced performance and outcomes. Once we have experienced the Flow state, we want to be in it more and more of the time.

Becoming conscious of the presence or absence of Flow in our lives allows us to take action and enhance it where needed. In this book, we will work with the lesser, larger, greater, and cosmic flows by awakening, encouraging, and deepening our understanding of them in order to improve our own health and quality of life. Craniosacral Chi Kung helps us become more conscious of Flow, and provides tools for cultivating more of it in our daily lives.

OPTIMAL FLOW

From a biomedical point of view, healthy flows fall within certain parameters, such as heart rate, breath rate, etc. It may be useful for us to be aware of these objective rates in order to monitor changes and to get a baseline about our health. Even with these objective measures, however, it is important to note that each person is unique: what is normal and healthy in one person may be an indicator of ill health for someone else.

Our subjective perception of flow rate is also a relevant consideration, however. Too much may feel overwhelming and taxing to our systems. When there is not enough movement, we feel stuck, congested, or stagnant. In this light, our relationship with Flow and our internal perception of it may be even more important than objective measures.

If you have ever watched someone surfing, you may notice that the critical difference between a poor ride and a great ride is not the objective speed of the wave, but whether or not the surfer is able to keep up with it. If surfers are not able to get up to speed with the wave, they get left behind without getting a ride at all. If they go too fast and get ahead of the wave, they fall out and get smashed by the wave as it breaks. But if they are in sync with the wave and are fluid and flexible in adjusting to it, they are carried effortlessly to new places. And if they are also able to relax and enjoy the ride, then they have the opportunity to have a peak experience.

Sensing Flow and Stagnation

In humans, Flow manifests in many ways. On the physical level, fluids such as blood, lymph, and cerebrospinal fluid (CSF) move through our bodies. Food and water move through our digestive and elimination systems, and oxygen is distributed from our lungs to the rest of the body. If these processes move too quickly we may hyperventilate or have diarrhea. When there is insufficient flow, we may notice issues such as edema or constipation.

Appropriate flow is also important on an emotional level. When we are emotionally volatile or overly reactive to a situation, our emotional flow may be too strong. And although we may not be used to thinking about it in this way, depression, resentment, or bitterness may be signs that our emotions have been stuck for a while, and that we need to encourage more emotional flow. When we are able to experience the entire spectrum of emotions, without becoming attached or mired in them, our emotional energy is flowing well.

It is also possible to notice the quality of our mental flow. On days when there is excessive flow, our thoughts may be racing, and we may find it difficult to focus or concentrate on a topic. At other times, our thoughts may seem to loop continuously. We may find it challenging to learn new things or we might be unreasonably resistant to modifying our current thoughts: these experiences are typical of insufficient mental fluidity. In contrast, when our mental energy is flowing in a balanced way, our thinking is clear, new creative thoughts arise easily, and we are easily able to accommodate new information.

The physical, emotional, and mental aspects of ourselves are interconnected, so it makes sense that too much or too little flow on one level affects the flow of the others. This strong interconnection also means that the benefits of harmonizing flow on one level will ripple out to the other levels, leading to greater health and harmony. And when our consciousness is flowing and up to speed, like being in sync with a wave, our spiritual self can have a peak experience.

CRANIOSACRAL METHODS OF TRACKING THE FLOW

Like Chi Kung, Craniosacral Work is all about Flow. Craniosacral practitioners develop finely-tuned abilities to sense where there is movement and where there is not movement in their clients. Many craniosacral techniques are designed to invite a return to Flow in areas that are restricted; other techniques encourage harmony among the various flows of the body.

Craniosacral practitioners assess Flow in terms of four basic characteristics: tempo, magnitude, balance, and quality (fig. 1.4). By asking a series of questions, such as those described below, practitioners can learn more about the specific flow with which they are in contact.

Tempo: What is the speed of the movement? This is generally measured in cycles per minute. Each type of flow in our body has a different tempo. The breath rate is different from the heart rate, for instance, and both of those are different from the rate at which cerebral spinal fluid moves through the system. The point here is to develop our awareness of the usual rate for each flow and encourage it to optimize.

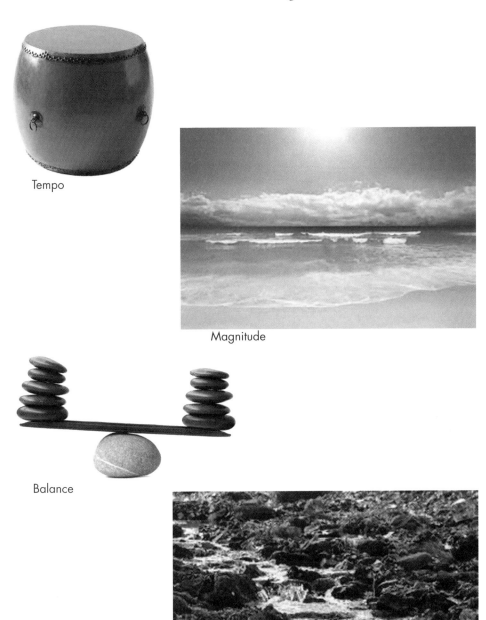

Tempo

Magnitude

Balance

Quality

Fig. 1.4. Four characteristics of Flow

Magnitude: What is the range of motion? How far do the structures move into flexion or extension? Is there full range of motion or are there some restrictions? Structures that are not able to move freely often block energy from circulating. Another way to frame this is to consider the volume or magnitude of the flow. Is it the merest trickle or a cascading stream? Typically, the greater the magnitude, the greater the vitality of the structure.

Balance: How symmetrical are the structures and how balanced is the motion? For example, is the right balanced with the left? Is flexion balanced with extension?

Quality: How would we describe the motion? What adjectives or adverbs would you use to describe what you are sensing? For example, does the movement feel sluggish, vibrant, smooth, or strong? This measure is subjective, but one of the most important for our internal perception of Flow.

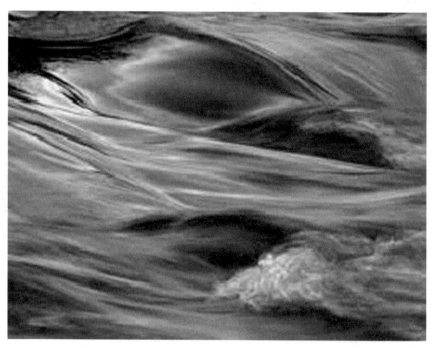

Fig. 1.5. Flowing over, around, and through obstacles

The Taoist way encourages us to learn about ourselves and take responsibility for our own self-care. Using the four measures above gives us a framework for better understanding the fluidity of our own systems. We have lived with ourselves for our entire lives, but may never before have paid attention to our internal rhythms in this way. Gaining a sense of our Flow is invaluable because it offers us more resources when we encounter challenging circumstances. Instead of tensing and becoming rigid, we become accustomed to relaxing, finding where there is Flow, and joining it (fig. 1.5). And when we are flowing in a balanced and harmonious way, we feel vibrant and vital.

BACK-TO-THE-BODY WISDOM

In modern society where the focus is often on mental skills, people can become disconnected from their physicality, creating imbalance by ignoring the valuable insights and different kinds of wisdom that the physical body offers. We often wait until we are in pain or experiencing illness before paying attention to our physical selves.

In the following chapters, we will show how Chi Kung practices help us improve Flow in every aspect of our lives. One of first benefits of these practices is increased awareness of the physical body. Tuning in to the physical body and feeling the dynamic changes as energy moves through it is what we call "back-to-the-body wisdom." It teaches us to listen to the whispers of disharmony before they become shouts.

Breath of Life

Food, water, and air are the basics we need to survive. Depending on our physical condition and external factors such as climate, we can go without food for several weeks and survive a few days without water if necessary. However, even the strongest and healthiest people can only live for a few minutes without air. Breath is life.

Respiration is an automatic function controlled by the respiratory center of the brain stem. Because it is automatic, we breathe without needing to consciously think about it; the *way* we breathe is often determined by patterns set when we were very young. It is estimated that over 90 percent of people begin to restrict their breathing before the age of five. Research studies link shallow breathing patterns to several physical and emotional disorders.

The good news is that breathing is also a voluntary function that can be consciously controlled: we can use mindful breathing practices to retrain our respiratory patterns and improve our health and well-being. As we return our breathing to its natural state, we reduce anxiety and stress, integrate our emotions, gain mental clarity, increase vitality, and regain a sense of peace and well-being. Breath work is a powerful tool for both internal and external development and that is why all wisdom traditions have breathing practices.

In Craniosacral Work, the term *Breath of Life* is used to describe a universal healing intelligence—like the Tao—that provides an organizing principle guiding us to health and healing. Dr. William Garner Sutherland, the father of cranial osteopathy, believed that the human system was more than simply bones, fluids, tissues, and biochemicals. Like the Taoist masters, he could sense subtle rhythmic wavelike fluctuations within the body. He understood that life-force energy manifests and expresses itself through tide-like movements, and that those movements are critical for health and healing. Craniosacral Work recognizes that there are many tides in the human body, but focuses on four in particular: the Cranial Wave, the Fluid Tide, the Long Tide, and the Long Wave. We will talk more about these fluid dynamics later in the book.

AWAKE, AWARE, APPRECIATE

Our spiritual journey is like our journey through a regular day. We start out asleep and then, when we awaken, our day begins. Once we are *awake,* we become conscious and curious about what is unfolding in our day and in our life. After being awake for a while (perhaps only a few moments or much longer), we actually become *aware* of ourselves

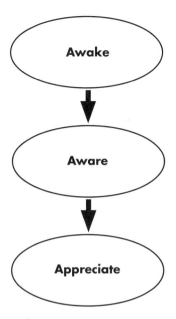

Fig. 1.6. Awake, Aware, Appreciate: a practice for
finding, generating, and sustaining Flow

and what is going on around us. Awareness enables us to be mindful
of our choices, our intentions, and the decisions that shape our day. By
realizing our part in how the day takes shape, we begin to *appreciate*
and therefore understand the purpose and benefits of our experiences,
and can place them into the context of our lives (fig. 1.6). When we do
practices such as the Inner Smile, we are deepening our understanding
of ourselves and the world in a profound way.

Throughout the rest of this book, as we play with the concepts of
Flow, we will use this process of awakening different aspects of Flow,
becoming aware of the Flow, and then learning to understand and
appreciate what Flow has to offer us.

ANCIENT TAOIST WISDOM ABOUT FLOW

Two thousand years ago, a Taoist master created a painting that illus-
trated the importance of Flow for life, relationships, and spiritual

development (fig. 1.7). Depicting a water wheel and irrigation, the painting is also a metaphor for the movement of fluids through our physical body and of chi through our energy body.

At the bottom of the painting, we see a boy and a girl stepping on a water wheel, which pumps water upward to irrigate the land. On the right side you can see the spine, which Taoists call the Celestial Pillar. The Celestial Pillar connects earth (the tailbone) and heaven (the head). When the spine is open and healthy and there is good flow along it, we can access the powers of both earth and heaven. This is why the ancient Taoists paid so much attention to the spine.

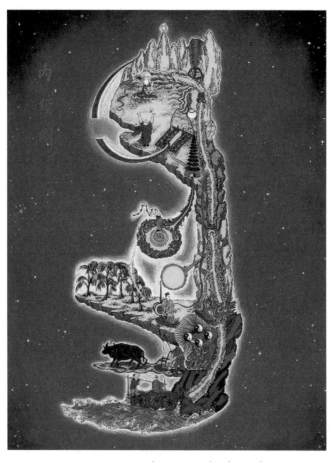

Fig. 1.7. Pumping the water wheel circulates
water to the top of the mountain.

The Three Gates of the Spine

For there to be good flow throughout the entire system, the three key gates of the spine must be open: the lower gate, the middle gate, and the upper gate (fig. 1.8).

The Lower Gate: Wei Lu Guan/Tailbone Pass

The lower gate is Wei Lu Guan or Tailbone Pass. It is located at the tailbone (coccyx) and sacrum. When this gate is closed then our sacrum is locked: we lose our connection with earth and may experience back pain. The ancient painting illustrates the stepping action of the water-wheel, which reflects the movement of the sacrum between the ilia. This motion of the sacrum creates a pumping action that sends cerebrospinal fluid through the central nervous system. At the same time, the pumping action opens the lower gate and tan tien, increasing Flow in the entire system and enhancing our physical vitality.

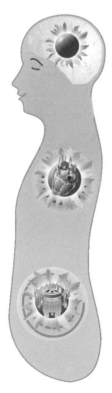

Fig. 1.8. Three gates of the spine

The Middle Gate: Jia Ji Guan/Squeeze the Spine Pass

The middle gate is Jia Ji Guan or Squeeze the Spine Pass. It is located in the area of the heart and lungs and is associated with the pumping motion of the diaphragm and heart. When this gate is open and energy is flowing smoothly through it, our emotional and mental bodies are clear and fluid. If this gate is blocked, however, our emotions may be stuck and our thinking muddy.

The Upper Gate: Yu Zhen Guan/Jade Pillow Pass

The upper gate is Yu Zhen Guan, or Jade Pillow Pass, which can be found at the base of the skull where the occiput meets the atlas. When energy cannot move smoothly through this gate, we may notice headaches and/ or difficulty accessing our spirituality. If this gate is clear, then we are connected with the cosmic Flow of heaven and the universe. When that occurs, we have access to spiritual wisdom and limitless Source.

Activating these three pumps enables us to generate energy and keep it flowing throughout our whole system. The upward movement of the waterwheel transforms *ching** (essence) into *chi* (energy), and chi into *shen* (spirit). The downward movement nourishes the chi and replenishes the ching. The navel fire helps transform water into steam (chi), which turns into rain and nourishes the whole organism. This continuous flow moves energy through the meridian pathways and the Microcosmic Orbit.

---

*The transliterated term *ching* is synonymous with the transliteration *jing* that appears in many discussions of Taoism.

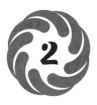

Awakening the
Major Pumps

While our bodies employ numerous systems for moving vital fluids and nutrients around, we can greatly improve all flows by focusing on the four major pumps, located in the three tan tiens (fig. 2.1):

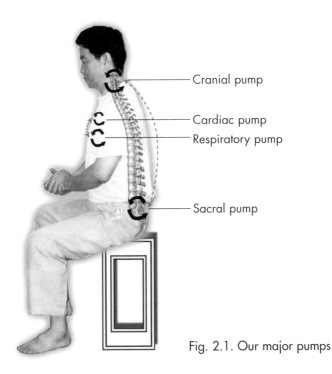

— Cranial pump

— Cardiac pump
— Respiratory pump

— Sacral pump

Fig. 2.1. Our major pumps

- The cranial pump of the upper tan tien
- The respiratory and cardiac pumps of the middle tan tien
- The sacral pump of the lower tan tien

All of these pumps are interconnected and interrelated, and are supported by Universal Healing Tao practices. In the next sections, we will look at the special interactions between the respiratory and cardiac pumps and the cranial and sacral pumps.

THE RESPIRATORY PUMP

The first thing we do when we are born is take a breath; this is also the last thing we do when we are making our transition out of this life.

Every wisdom tradition includes breath work. It is one of the most valuable tools for connecting our physical body with our energy body. It is always available and requires no fancy equipment. Since we breathe from the moment we are born until we die, we have the opportunity to practice throughout our entire life. Yet, although we breathe all the time, often we are not conscious of much of what is happening during the process.

Many of us tend to associate breathing with the lungs. However, in reality, it is the diaphragm—the large flat muscle that separates the heart, lungs, and ribs from the abdomen—that is doing much of the work (fig. 2.2). As we inhale, the diaphragm moves downward. This stretches the lungs and causes them to expand, drawing in air. As we exhale, the diaphragm relaxes and moves upward into the chest cavity. As the diaphragm pushes against the lungs, they expel air, which exits through the nose and mouth.

Taoist breathing exercises emphasize the movement of the abdomen, which can control the diaphragm to activate the respiratory pump. For example, reverse breathing contracts the abdomen on inhalation. This lowers the diaphragm, increasing pressure in the abdomen and packing energy from the breath into the tissues, organs, and spine. On exhalation, the diaphragm relaxes and moves upward as the stomach relaxes

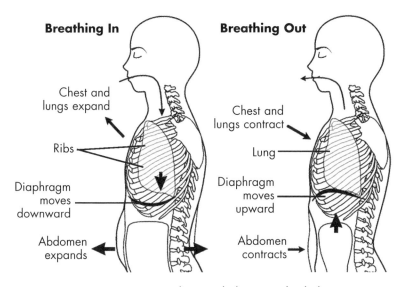

Fig. 2.2. Respiratory pump during inhalation and exhalation

outward. As the pressure in the abdomen is released, the energy flows outward to wherever we direct it with our intention.

Awakening the Breath of Life

Breathing is both a subconscious and conscious activity. We don't need to think about breathing in order for it to happen, but if we are conscious of it, we can modify our breathing and create significant changes to our physical, emotional, mental, and energetic health. The exercises below introduce basic Taoist breathing techniques for awakening the flow of the breath.

With each breath, imagine you are filling a glass with water. As water pours into the glass, it fills from the bottom up. When you empty the glass, water pours out from the top down. Similarly, feel air filling your lower abdomen first as you inhale, then the upper abdomen, and finally your chest, until you have taken a deep full breath. And as you exhale, imagine the air leaving from the upper part of your chest first, then the middle, then the lower abdomen.

In these exercises, both inhalation and exhalation are done through the nose; the tongue is placed on the roof of the mouth. Ideally, inhalation and exhalation are of equal length and the breath is slow, smooth, silent, and effortless.

Deep breathing helps to oxygenate the system, release adhesions, massage our internal organs, and increase circulation throughout the entire body. When our organs adhere to each other and lose their range of motion, our blood flow is reduced. This blocks energy flow. If the energy block continues, we become more vulnerable to chronic disease. Deep breathing is one of the best ways that we can promote energy flow, blood flow, and overall health.

Natural or Abdominal Breathing

1. As you inhale, allow your lower belly to expand in all directions like a balloon (fig. 2.3).
2. When your lungs are full, exhale slowly, allowing your belly to move back toward the spine as it gently contracts.
3. Continue for 18 full cycles of breath.
4. Repeat another 18 times while gradually increasing your speed until your diaphragm is moving vigorously and the breath is like a bellows. This builds energy in the lower tan tien, igniting more activity in this core area.

In addition to the general benefits of deep breathing, natural breathing helps to reduce blood pressure, slow the heart rate, and eliminate toxins more quickly.

Advanced Variation

Once you have become familiar with natural breathing, or if you are an advanced practitioner, you can press your sacrum backward on inhalation and tuck it under during exhalation. This will increase the benefits of the exercise.

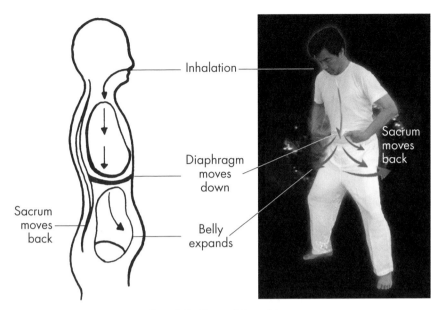

Inhalation

Diaphragm moves down

Sacrum moves back

Belly expands

Sacrum moves back

Fig. 2.3. Natural Breathing

 Reverse Breathing

In addition to the general benefits of deep breathing, reverse breathing is used to build chi in the kidneys and draw it deeply into the tissues and bones, strengthening the immune system (see fig. 2.4 on page 30). It is also good for toning the abdominal muscles and increasing lung capacity. Reverse breathing contributes to our core energy foundation and supports the heart.

1. During inhalation, draw your belly back toward the spine.
2. At the same time, contract and draw the Hui Yin/perineum point upward. (The Hui Yin/perineum is behind the sexual organs and in front of the anus.)
3. During exhalation, allow the belly to release outward slowly, expanding like a balloon in all directions.
4. Continue for 18 full cycles of breath, then repeat for another 18 cycles, gradually increasing your speed so that your abdomen expands firmly with each exhalation.

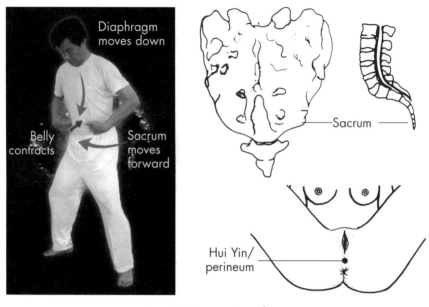

Fig. 2.4. Reverse Breathing

⊙ *Advanced Variation*

Once you have become familiar with reverse breathing, or if you are an advanced practitioner, you can tuck your sacrum during inhalation and press it backward on exhalation to increase the benefits of the exercise.

THE CARDIAC PUMP

The cardiac pump circulates blood throughout the body. About the size of a fist, the heart consists of four chambers: the left and right atria above, and the left and right ventricles below (fig. 2.5). The atria collect blood and the ventricles distribute it. The heart takes in deoxygenated blood through the veins, then sends it to the lungs for oxygenation before pumping it back to the rest of the body through the arteries.

Heartbeat

The sinoatrial node (SA node), located in the right atrium, is the heart's pacemaker—the initiator of the heartbeat. Electrical impulses from the

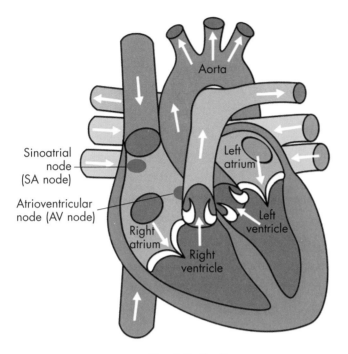

Fig. 2.5. Cardiac pump

SA node cause the atria to contract and the ventricles to fill with blood. The electrical impulse then continues to the ventricles, which contract and send blood outward. The SA node pacemaker initiates the beat, but the autonomic nervous system determines the rate of the beat and the strength of the contraction.

When the sympathetic (fight-or-flight) nervous system is active, the heart rate increases and the heart beats more forcefully. The parasympathetic (rest and rejuvenation) system slows the heart rate and reduces the force of the heart's contraction.

Science has demonstrated that hearts, even if removed from the body, will continue beating for a long time if given sufficient nutrients.[1] They have a will and life of their own. Studies also show that hearts will entrain with each other and begin to beat in synchrony when in close proximity.[2] So the SA node not only sets the tempo for each individual but can also influence the cadence of other people and even entire groups.

Heart Work

The average heart beats 72 times per minute, pumping approximately 70 ml (2.4 ounces) of blood with each beat. The typical adult heart beats over 100,000 times daily and around 3 million times each year: this translates into 5 liters (1.3 gallons) each minute, 7,200 liters (1,900 gallons) per day, and 2.6 million liters (nearly 700,000 gallons) per year. By age 70, our hearts will have beaten 2.5 billion times and pumped an impressive 184 million liters (48 million gallons) of blood. This is even more remarkable because it does so without even a minute of rest.

That is a lot of work. In some wisdom traditions, it is said that we are born with a set number of heartbeats for our life. If we lead a hectic stressful life—one in which our heart is often racing—then we will use up those heartbeats faster and therefore die earlier. Although it temporarily increases our heart rate, physical exercise is good for our health over the long run because it strengthens the heart. A stronger heart does not need to beat as often to pump the blood and therefore exercise reduces our average heart rate.

According to the American Institute of Stress, as much as 90 percent of all visits to primary care physicians are related to stress.[3] Therefore, if we follow meditation and Chi Kung practices that reduce stress, calm our nervous system, and slow our heart rate, it is likely that we will live longer and healthier lives.

Heart Power

The heart creates the strongest electromagnetic field in the body, generating an electrical field sixty times larger than the brain's and a magnetic field five thousand times larger (fig. 2.6). Neurocardiologists estimate that 60–65 percent of heart cells are neurons rather than muscle: their research shows that the heart's nervous system works similarly to the brain and could be considered to be another independent brain.[4] Scientists can measure the energy of the heart from at least five feet away.

Studies by the HeartMath Institute show that the heart's electro-

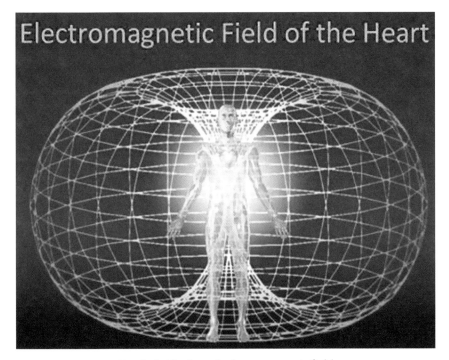

Fig. 2.6. The heart's electromagnetic field

magnetic field, as well as the rhythmic patterns of our heartbeat, have a powerful influence on our physical health, mental clarity, emotional state, and interactions with others.[5] Since it is our link to Source, we must connect with the heart to access our full power.

Seat of the Soul

In Taoism, the heart is where our Original Spirit resides. The heart connects us with the Source, the Supreme Creator, and enables us to both experience unconditional love and to radiate it to our communities.

The Upanishads say that in the core of the heart is the support and foundation of the universe, and in the middle of that core is a great fire that warms everything. The source of the fire is very small, but very powerful, and it is the seat of our soul. The essential core of the heart—and the seat of the soul—is the sinoatrial node.

The sinoatrial node is not only influenced by our physical and emotional state, but is also deeply attuned to life itself and affected directly by Source. When working with the heart, focusing our awareness specifically on the SA node enhances the effect of connecting with the heart's own light and essence, and allows us to access the even greater light of Source more easily.

The SA node's location, two finger-widths to the right of center, places it in a region known as our secret esoteric heart. In Ecclesiastes, the Bible says that the heart of the wise inclines to the right and in fact, our hearts tilt rightward, in the direction of the SA node.

Awakening the Heart

In Chinese medicine, the Heart governs the body and is the most powerful of the organ meridians. As the commander, it influences all the other systems. The next exercise, Tapping into the Heart, helps us to connect with the heart more deeply and increase our awareness of it.

Tapping into the Heart

1. Sitting comfortably, place one or both hands on your heart.
2. Begin deep natural breathing.
3. Bringing your attention to your heart, allow your focus to sink more deeply into it, while lightening any physical pressure you might be creating with your hand.
4. Notice that the lighter your touch, the more you can sense.
5. Imagine yourself connecting with the sinoatrial node in the top right quadrant of your heart.
6. Sense into the spark that ignites the heart. Feel the awesome power of that creative impulse as it awakens.
7. As the heart lights up, sense its connection with Source and love, joy, and happiness.

HOW THE CARDIAC AND
RESPIRATORY PUMPS WORK TOGETHER

Now that you have awakened and increased your awareness of both your breath and your heart, you can begin to increase your appreciation of the interaction between the respiratory and cardiac pumps (fig. 2.7).

In order to live, we need both blood and oxygen. The heart and lungs work closely together to deliver these nutrients to all the cells in the body. In the heart, the atria receive blood and the ventricles distribute it. The right atrium collects oxygen-poor blood and sends it to the right ventricle, which pumps it into the lungs. The lungs oxygenate the

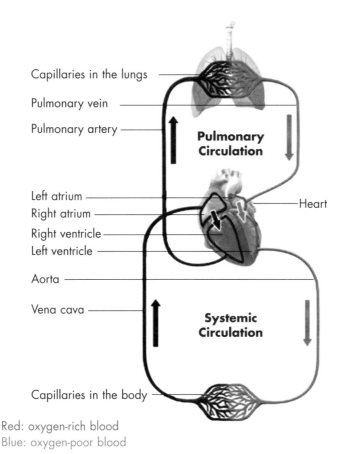

Fig. 2.7. Flow of oxygen and blood

blood via inhalation, remove the carbon dioxide through exhalation, and then pump the oxygen-rich blood back to the left atrium. The left atrium sends the oxygenated blood to the left ventricle for distribution to the rest of the body. As blood flows around the body bringing nutrients to the cells, oxygen becomes depleted. This oxygen-poor blood then returns to the heart, which pumps it back to the lungs to begin the process again.

This interaction between heart and lungs delivers oxygen and nutrients throughout the body, while simultaneously carrying away carbon dioxide and other wastes to be removed by the lungs, liver, and kidneys. The heart and vascular system influence respiration by controlling the amount of carbon dioxide in the bloodstream. Sensors in the brain, aorta, and carotid arteries monitor oxygen and carbon dioxide levels in the blood. Higher carbon dioxide levels signal the lungs to breathe more deeply to release the excess carbon dioxide, and the heart to pump harder. In the same way, low carbon dioxide levels in the blood signal breathing to slow temporarily while oxygen in the blood is delivered to the cells of the body. Low blood oxygen saturation raises blood pressure as the heart and lungs work to increase oxygen in the body.

Balancing the Heart and Lungs

When we think about breathing, we tend to think about taking in oxygen to nourish our cells, but releasing the right amount of carbon dioxide (CO_2) is also vitally important. Our hectic lifestyles and fast pace cause many of us to breathe more quickly and shallowly than is optimal. It also means that our inhalations tend to be much longer than our exhalations. A short exhalation means we are not releasing enough CO_2, which impacts our oxygen/CO_2 balance and causes acid and toxins to accumulate in our blood, tissues, and bones. With many people, the bottom quarter of the lungs remains filled with carbon dioxide, which reduces their ability to take a deep, full inhalation.

We need to clear the refrigerator (lungs) and dump the garbage (CO_2) to make room for new food (oxygen). The Chi Kung Breath of

Life exercise helps to regulate breathing and improve our oxygen/CO_2 balance, leading to more energy, improved mental capabilities, and less stress on our systems.

Chi Kung Breath of Life

1. Sit comfortably with your hands on your lap. Smile.
2. With your palms facing upward, inhale as you stretch your arms outward and overhead to gather energy.
3. Press your palms upward and extend your thumbs outward and up to the sky to invite the Lung meridian to open more fully (fig. 2.8).

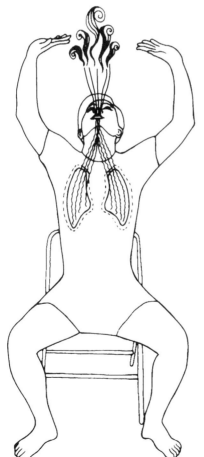

Fig. 2.8. Breath of Life exercise

4. Exhale with the sound "sss-s-s-s-s-s" to clear the lungs, release CO_2, and make room for more oxygen.
5. On your next inhalation, relax and smile. As you inhale, turn the palms downward and allow them to float down to your lap.
6. Exhale smoothly and fully through the nose while enjoying the clearing.
7. Let the energy flow through your entire body.
8. Repeat 9 times.

Notice how your energy has increased and your emotions have calmed after this exercise.

⟳ Variation

If you do not have space, or do not feel comfortable lifting your hands above your head, you can perform the following variation of the Breath of Life exercise.

1. Place your hands under your ribcage and take a small inhalation, letting your stomach expand.
2. On exhalation, lean forward slightly and bring your belly toward your spine.
3. Let the energy flow through your entire body.
4. Repeat 9 times.

Connecting Heart and Breath

In addition to the close functional interactions between heart and lungs in managing the flow of oxygen and blood through the body, there is also a link through the connective tissue. The mediastinum is a web of soft connective tissue that sits between the lungs, enclosing the heart along with the other organs and tissues of the chest (fig. 2.9). Running all the way to the cranial base, this tissue is what connects the head, heart, lungs, and diaphragm.

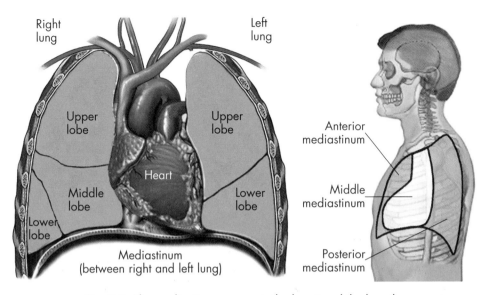

Fig. 2.9. The mediastinum connects the heart and the breath.

Another anatomical connection between heart and breath is that the heart sits on the central tendon of the diaphragm. Heaviness or stress in the heart is therefore communicated to the lungs via increased pressure on the diaphragm and tension in the mediastinum. Likewise, any practices that we do to relax and open the breath will simultaneously aid our hearts.

We can directly experience the relationship between the heart and lungs in their automatic synchronization. When our breath quickens, so does our heart rate. When we slow our breath, our heart slows as well. The smoother and deeper our breath, the more rhythmic and resonant our heartbeat. Without conscious intent or action, what affects one affects the other.

Breathing into the Heart

1. At the start of your practice, notice your heart rate.
2. Begin natural breathing. As you relax and settle into the practice, your breath will begin to slow and lengthen.

3. As your breathing slows, notice that your heart rate naturally begins to slow as well.

4. Begin to imagine that you are breathing into your heart (fig. 2.10). Feel the connection between the heart and breath increasing.

5. With every inhalation, draw the qualities of calmness and peace directly into your heart.

6. With every exhalation, let go of any tension and feel it dissipate.

7. After a few cycles of breathing, notice that both your breathing and your heart rate have slowed and become calmer.

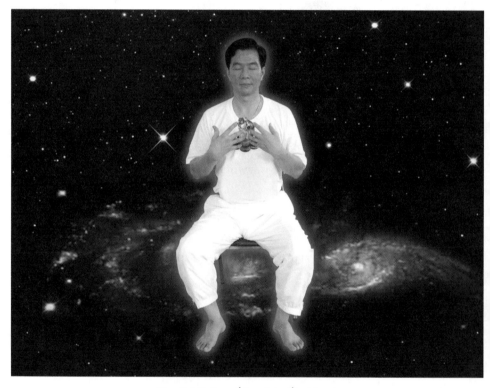

Fig. 2.10. Breathing into the Heart

In addition to the cardiac and respiratory pumps, the cranial and sacral pumps are the other two major pumps of the body. These pumps relate to each other through the flow of cerebrospinal fluid (CSF), the movement of the bones, and the elastic tissue of the dural tube.

THE CRANIAL PUMP

The cranium or skull has two main parts: the viscerocranium includes the fourteen facial bones while the neurocranium consists of the eight bones that enclose the brain (fig. 2.11). As all the bones of the skull and their surrounding membranes move and flex, they pump cerebrospinal fluid around the brain and through the spinal cord. Although all of the twenty-two bones of the cranium are moving, the cranial pump is most often associated with the occiput, the large bone at the base of the skull.

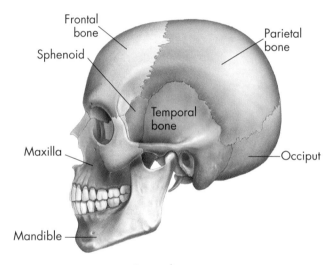

Frontal bone

Parietal bone

Sphenoid

Temporal bone

Maxilla

Occiput

Mandible

Fig. 2.11. The cranium

THE SACRAL PUMP

The sacrum is a triangular-shaped bone that sits between the two hip bones at the base of the spine (see fig. 2.12 on page 42). It connects with the lumbar spine above it and the coccyx below. The sacrum is composed of five vertebrae that begin to fuse when we are in our mid-teens; by our mid-thirties they have typically become one bone (see fig. 2.13 on page 42).

The forward and backward movements (flexion and extension) of the sacrum also pump CSF through the nervous system.

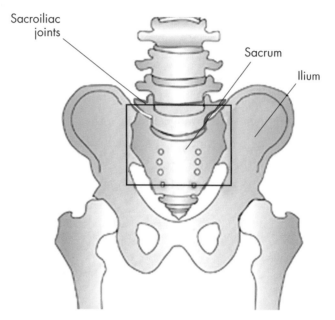

Fig. 2.12. The sacrum

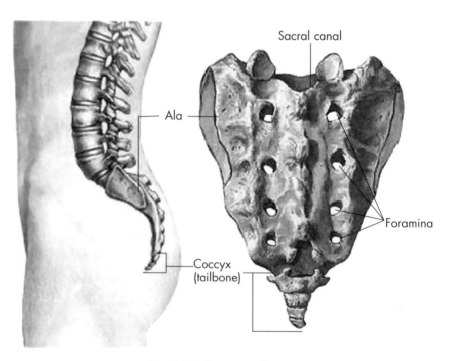

Fig. 2.13. Sacrum and coccyx

THE CRANIOSACRAL SYSTEM

Together, the brain and the spinal cord comprise the central nervous system. The spinal cord is a bundle of nerves whose main job is to transmit motor and sensory information between the brain and the rest of the body. The spinal cord is surrounded by a sheath of membrane called the dura mater or "tough mother." Like a tough mother, the dura mater's role is to protect the vulnerable spinal cord.

The dura mater extends from the head to the coccyx, attaching to the skeleton at the occiput (the base of the skull), the axis (C2), the sacrum (S2), and the coccyx (tailbone) (fig. 2.14). In between these attachments, the dura mater floats freely. Flexible and elastic, it stretches, compresses, and twists as we move. These shifts alter the shape of the

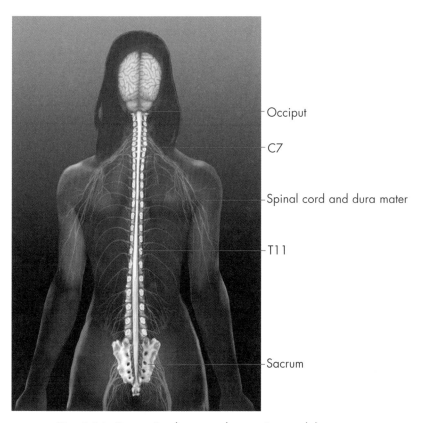

Occiput

C7

Spinal cord and dura mater

T11

Sacrum

Fig. 2.14. Connection between the cranium and the sacrum

spinal cord and brain as well as causing changes in the intensity, frequency, and amount of nerve flow.

Since its job is to protect the spinal cord, the dura (think "durable") is tough and thick. If the dura contracts—from stress and tension for example—it can even restrict the movement of the brain within the skull and spine, causing headaches, sciatica, and low back pain. That is why many Taoist practices work to increase fluidity of the spine and surrounding structures.

Because the bones of the sacrum and cranium (specifically the occiput) are connected by the elastic tissue of the dura mater, movement at one end causes the other end to move as well. Together, they create a semi-closed hydraulic pumping system called the craniosacral system, which circulates the cerebrospinal fluid. When healthy, the craniosacral system has a regular rhythm that balances and energizes the entire nervous system, benefitting our physical, emotional, and mental health.

Cerebrospinal Fluid

Cerebrospinal fluid (CSF) is a clear, colorless body fluid that flows primarily in and around the brain and spinal cord (fig. 2.15). Produced largely within the ventricles of the brain, CSF then circulates out to the rest of the nervous system and is eventually absorbed into the blood-stream. At any one time, there is about 150 ml of CSF circulating through our system. With an average daily production of ~500 ml, it is completely replenished slightly more than three times every day in a healthy adult.

CSF plays several critical roles in our health and wellness.

- **Nurturing:** As it flows around the brain and spinal cord and is absorbed back into the bloodstream, CSF provides nutrients and removes waste products.
- **Uplifting:** With the specific gravity of saltwater, CSF allows the brain to float buoyantly in its own private ocean so that it is not damaged at the base by the pressure of its own weight.
- **Protecting:** CSF offers a protective shock absorber from impacts

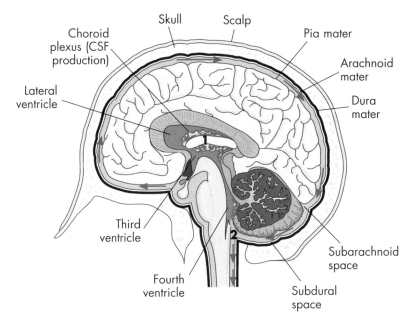

1. CSF is produced by the choroid plexus of each ventricle.
2. CSF flows through the ventricles and into the subarachnoid space as well as through the spinal cord.

Fig. 2.15. Cerebrospinal fluid is produced within the brain's ventricles and flows through the brain and down the spinal cord.

to the head and acts as an immunological buffer that reduces infections.

- **Adjusting:** The flow of CSF helps to adjust intracranial blood volume and pressure, preventing ischemia (reduced blood flow) and encouraging blood profusion.
- **Connecting:** The CSF transports hormones, neuropeptides, information, and energy to remote sites. It is the most conductive fluid in the body.

Connection and Conductivity

In craniosacral work, it is useful to highlight CSF's role in transporting neuropeptide messenger molecules and electrolytes throughout the body. Much of the communication throughout our body is done via electrical impulses, and CSF is an important conductor. Our body needs the information traveling to and from the brain in order to function. If the CSF is not flowing well, then our personal information intranet—and therefore our internal self-correcting mechanisms—cannot do their jobs. Insufficient CSF flow may lead to sensory, motor, or neurological problems.

CSF also contains the greatest concentration of neuropeptides, which coordinate body functions (such as digestion, elimination, and respiration) and play an important role in our mental-emotional balance. Although neuropeptides are present in the blood, they primarily circulate through our body via the cerebrospinal fluid, where they play a critical part in cellular functioning. Neuropeptides determine the health of our cells, which in turn determines our overall health.

Dr. Andrew Taylor Still, the founder of osteopathy, referred to CSF as one of the highest known elements of the human body. Dr. Randolph Stone, creator of polarity therapy, said that the soul swims in cerebrospinal fluid and that CSF is the liquid medium for the Breath of Life. In the Taoist cosmology, CSF is perceived as the fluid with the highest vibration in the physical body.

As Above, So Below

The double pumping mechanism of the cranial and sacral pumps bathes the central nervous system with CSF, transporting the neuropeptides and electrolytes that keep our cells functioning and communication flowing. To do this, the cranium and sacrum must move constantly, fluidly, and rhythmically. Many of the Universal Healing Tao practices are well-designed to build and amplify the connection between the head and the sacrum. Craniosacral movement is naturally refined and subtle. It is powerfully effective without being overt; most people are unaware that this critical inner Flow exists. When we do exercises like stretching the lower back, or tilting and rotating the hips and the sacrum, we gently augment the natural flow, taking advantage of this anatomical connection between the upper and lower tan tiens or heaven and earth. In Craniosacral Work, this connection is called the Core Link.

Returning to the ancient Taoist picture of the water wheel, we can think of it as a twenty-four-story high-rise apartment building. The twenty-four stories represent the twenty-four vertebrae of the lumbar (5), thoracic (12), and cervical spine (7). If the pumping system is not powerful enough, the upper levels do not receive sufficient liquid for drinking, cooking, or cleaning. Without this precious fluid, the health of the inhabitants then suffers and the building falls into disrepair. The purpose of many of the Chi Kung exercises is to open the gates and activate the pumps so that our essential fluids, especially cerebrospinal fluid, can circulate freely between our head and tail. This helps us maintain and improve our health.

OPENING THE SACRAL PUMP

Many Chi Kung practitioners find it challenging to feel the movement of the sacrum because they confuse it with the movement of the waist and hips. The following exercises are designed to build more discernment by helping you to feel the differences among these areas.

Tip: Take Your Time. The great sage Lao Tzu observed that nature does not hurry, yet everything is accomplished. When we zip along the highway going 70 mph, we are going too quickly to be able to notice much. If we drive along the regular streets at 5 mph, we have more opportunity to notice all the interesting things that are happening along our journey. The slower you do these exercises, the easier it is to notice what is going on.

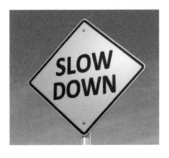

Fig. 2.16. Slow down.

Opening the Waist

1. Place your hands on your waist.
2. Slowly begin to rotate your waist, allowing the upper body to move as well—as if you are playing with a large hula hoop (fig. 2.17).
3. Circle 9 times in a clockwise direction, then 9 times in a counter-clockwise direction.

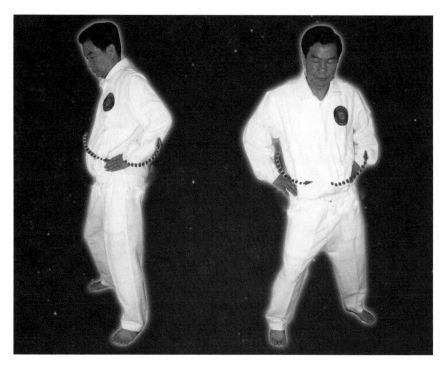

Fig. 2.17. Opening the Waist

 ## Opening the Hips

1. Bring your hands to your hip bones (fig. 2.18).
2. Keeping your upper body relatively still and your head above your feet, rotate your hips slowly in a clockwise direction 9 times.
3. Then, reverse the rotation by moving your hips 9 times in a counter-clockwise direction.

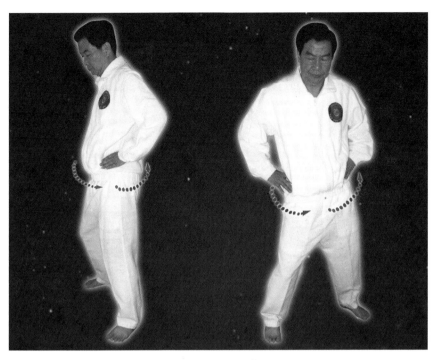

Fig. 2.18. Opening the Hips

Rotating the Sacrum

1. Touch the thumb and index fingers of one hand to those of the other hand with the index fingers pointing down.
2. With your hands in this position, place them behind you on your sacrum. Notice that your thumbs and index fingers outline the triangular edges of the sacral bone (fig. 2.19).

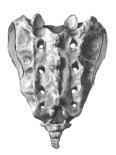

Fig. 2.19. The sacrum has a triangular shape.

3. Bring your attention to the sacrum.

4. Keeping your hips still, invite the sacrum to rotate slowly 9 times in one direction (fig. 2.20).

5. Reverse the direction and rotate the sacrum 9 times in the opposite direction.

Only the sacrum—not the hips or waist—should move. Its movements will be small and subtle.

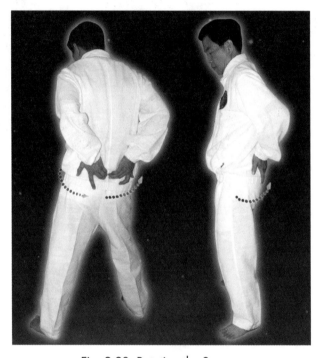

Fig. 2.20. Rotating the Sacrum

Awakening the Sacral Pump

1. Stand comfortably with your feet shoulder-width apart. Place the palms of your hands on your sacrum (fig. 2.21).

2. Slowly begin to tilt your pelvis forward into flexion by tucking your tailbone.

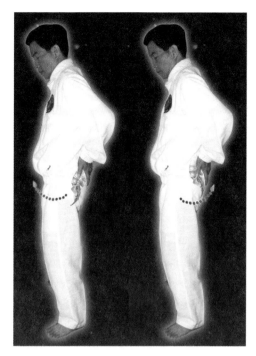

Fig. 2.21. Awakening the Sacral Pump

3. Next, press your sacrum backward into extension.
4. Alternate tucking and pressing your sacrum backward and forward in a gentle swinging motion.

Rocking your sacrum activates the sacral pump. This movement of the sacrum is foundational for Tai Chi, Tan Tien Chi Kung, and Iron Shirt Chi Kung. It is also an excellent exercise to relax the lower back and relieve stress.

The Sacral Nerves

The sacral nerves pass through the sacral foramen—the four small holes on each side of the sacrum. These nerves are responsible for sensory perception and motor function in the lower extremities. These nerve fibers are also related to the colon, rectum, bladder, genitals, and the parasympathetic nervous system.

Western medicine uses sacral nerve stimulation to treat bladder issues such as urgency, frequency, and incontinence, as well as constipation, pressure ulcers, and issues with the pelvic floor. With sacral nerve stimulation therapy, a small neurotransmitter is implanted in the buttock. It sends electrical impulses to the sacral nerves that affect the bladder and sphincter.

In the United States, millions of people report sciatic or lower back pain each year. The sciatic nerve is the longest nerve in the body, extending from the lower spine down to the legs. It provides feeling and movement in the hamstrings, lower legs, and feet. When the sciatic nerve is irritated, people often experience burning, tingling, or numbness in the lower back, buttocks, and legs. The Taoist practices above help to bring increased circulation and flow to the sacral areas which can help to prevent and relieve sciatic nerve dysfunction as well as soothe the nervous system.

Filling the Sacral Pump

1. Rub your hands briskly. Invite universal chi to fill them.
2. Now place your warm hands on your sacrum and gently palpate until you can feel the four small holes (sacral foramen) on the right side of the sacrum and the four foramen on the left (fig. 2.22).

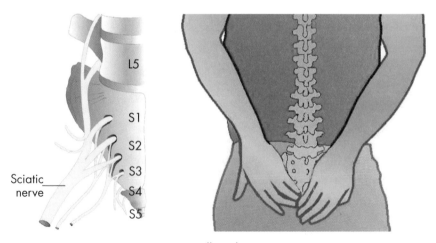

Fig. 2.22. Filling the sacrum

3. Bring your attention to these holes and allow chi to flow into them and fill them.

Opening the Cranial Pump

In modern society, many of us spend several hours a day leaning forward while working on the computer or driving. When the head is not in good alignment, the neck muscles become tense trying to hold it up. Since the weight of the average adult human head is 8–12 pounds, that is a lot of weight for the neck to support (fig. 2.23).

Additionally, the neck is one of the most vulnerable parts of the human body. Because we instinctively try to protect our necks when we feel threatened, we automatically tense our neck and shoulders as a defensive mechanism in times of stress. Chronic stress leads to chronic neck tension. Over time, that tension can restrict the cranial pump from optimal functioning.

To open up your cranial pump and soften your neck and shoulders, try the following simple exercises.

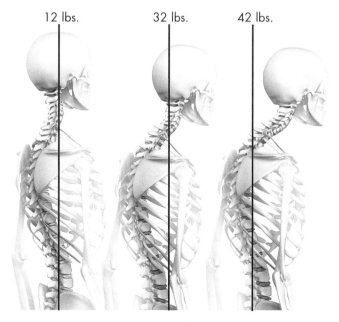

Fig. 2.23. Neck tension

Rocking the Neck

1. Tip your chin gently down toward your chest (fig. 2.24).
2. Take a full breath in and out while your neck relaxes in this position.
3. Return your head to neutral, then tilt your chin up to the sky.
4. Take a full breath in and out to allow your neck to relax and open.
5. Return your head to center and continue for 9 cycles.

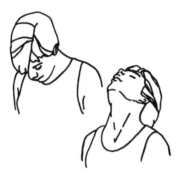

Fig. 2.24. Rocking the Neck

 Bending the Neck

1. Bring your right ear to your right shoulder while keeping your left shoulder relaxed and down (fig. 2.25).
2. Bring your head back to center and pause.
3. Invite your left ear to move toward your left shoulder while keeping the right shoulder relaxed and down.
4. Return to center and continue for a total of 9 cycles.

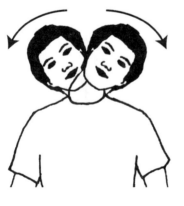

Fig. 2.25. Bending the Neck

Rotating the Neck

1. Relax your shoulders.
2. Turn your chin to the right as far as it will comfortably go. This movement will rotate the neck on its axis (fig. 2.26).
3. Return to center and pause.
4. Turn your chin to the left to the comfortable limit of its range.
5. Return to center and complete 9 cycles.

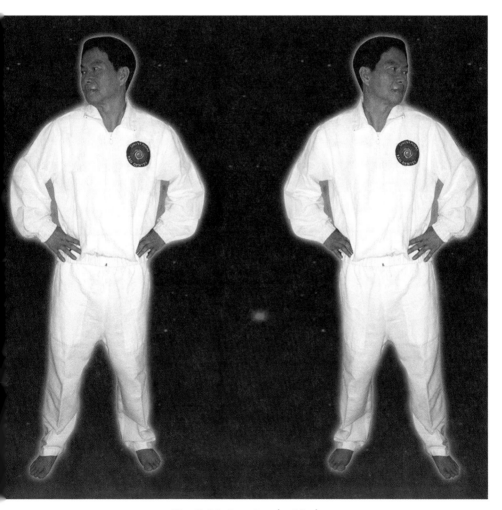

Fig. 2.26. Rotating the Neck

Rolling the Neck

1. Slowly and gently roll your neck clockwise. Let your chin lead as if it is moving around the face of a clock (fig. 2.27).
2. Do 9 complete circles.
3. Repeat in the counterclockwise direction for another 9 circles.

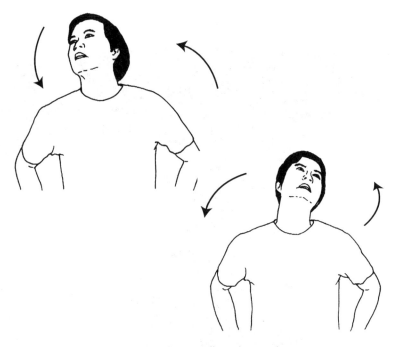

Fig. 2.27. Rolling the Neck

 ## Activating the Cranial Pump

1. Stand comfortably with your back against a wall (fig. 2.28).
2. Relax your shoulders and let them round forward slightly.
3. Tuck your chin and gently press the back of your head and neck behind you toward the wall, taking your neck into flexion.
4. Release and relax the chin, letting it lift up and back into extension as far as is comfortable without hitting the wall behind you.

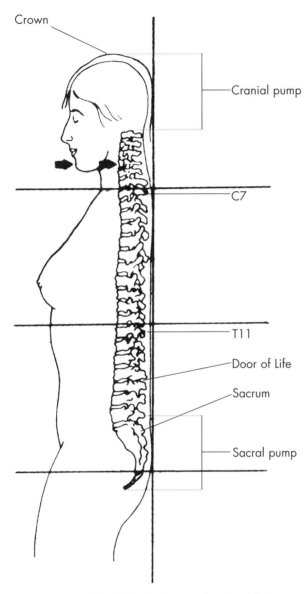

Crown

Cranial pump

C7

T11

Door of Life

Sacrum

Sacral pump

Fig. 2.28. Activating the Cranial Pump

Do 3 sets of 3 cycles of flexion and extension, pausing between sets to sense the increased movement through the cranial pump. You may also notice additional changes throughout the upper back, mid-back, lower back, and sacral pump.

AWAKENING THE CORE LINK
BETWEEN THE CRANIUM AND SACRUM

Earlier in this chapter we mentioned the soft tissue dura mater connection between the cranium and the sacrum—the Core Link. For good flow in the physical body, there must be good connection and communication between heaven (the cranium) and earth (the sacrum). Spinal Cord Breathing is one of the best ways to awaken this connection and keep it healthy.

Spinal Cord Breathing enlivens the spine, promotes good range of motion and flexibility, activates the cranial and sacral pumps, and enhances the flow of cerebral spinal fluid. It also helps to relax the back muscles so meditation is comfortable, and increases the flow of chi through the spine.

In modern life, many people work at a desk and sit for many hours a day. Additionally, many people also sit watching television or playing on the internet once they are home. So much sitting hinders the motion of the sacrum and reduces Flow. Spinal Cord Breathing is a great way to counteract the ill effects of prolonged sitting.

 ## Spinal Cord Breathing

1. Stand with your feet shoulder-width apart and your knees slightly bent.
2. Relax, and begin to notice how you feel.
3. Begin natural breathing.
4. On your next inhalation, keeping your elbows bent and your fingers toward the sky, bring your arms level with your shoulders and pulled slightly back. Gently tilt your sacrum backward, arching your spine (fig. 2.29). Open your chest and allow the rib cage to expand, activating the thymus and adrenal glands. Allow your head to drop backward and allow your jaw to soften.
5. As you exhale, tilt your sacrum forward, tucking your tailbone and

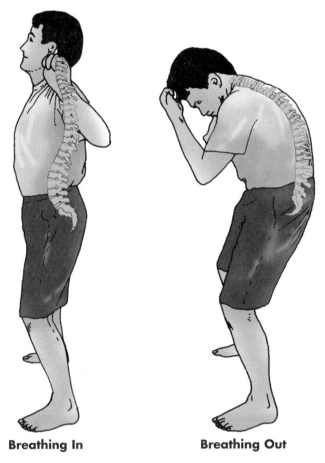

Breathing In   **Breathing Out**

Fig. 2.29. Spinal Cord Breathing

rounding your spine as if curling into a ball. Bring your elbows together in front of your chest, and let your chin drop toward your chest as you lightly clench your teeth.

6. Repeat 9 or 18 times, then return your head and spine to neutral and rest.

In addition to Spinal Cord Breathing, the Crane, Turtle, and Wagging the Dragon's Tail exercises are also helpful in waking up the Core Link. All of these exercises are best done standing, but they can be done sitting if necessary.

Crane

1. Stand with your feet shoulder-width apart and your knees bent to allow the energy to flow freely. Rest your palms easily on your thighs (fig. 2.30).
2. Inhale slowly and evenly.
3. As you exhale, lean as far forward as you can, letting your chin lead your movement.
4. When you reach your limit, keep your chin extended and let it dive downward as far as you can.
5. Tuck your chin to your chest and roll upward until your spine is straight again. Allow your chin to relax.
6. Repeat 9 times, then rest.
7. Feel the sensation of movement along the Core Link.

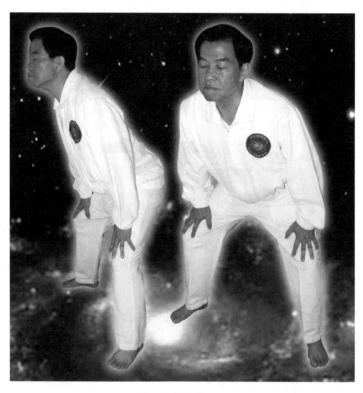

Fig. 2.30. Crane

Turtle

1. Stand with your feet shoulder-width apart and your knees bent to allow the energy to flow freely. Rest your palms easily on your thighs.
2. Inhale slowly and evenly.
3. As you exhale, tuck your chin to your chest and follow it downward, rounding your spine until you reach your limit (fig. 2.31).
4. Extend your chin forward and follow it upward in a gentle circle until your spine is straight and your head is over your hips.
5. Repeat 9 times, then rest, feeling the movement in your Core Link.

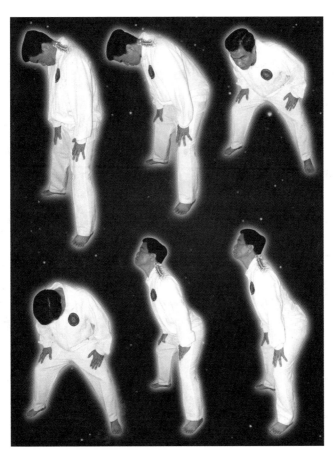

Fig. 2.31. Turtle

Wagging the Dragon's Tail

1. Sit down and smile to your spine.
2. Begin to gently rock your spine left and right, like a dragon wagging its tail (fig. 2.32).
3. Feel each vertebra, from the lumbar through the thoracic and then to the cervical spine. Feel your spine opening in a lateral direction.

Rocking side-to-side in this way creates a vibration throughout the whole spine, allowing energy to move freely through the entire back and opening up the Core Link.

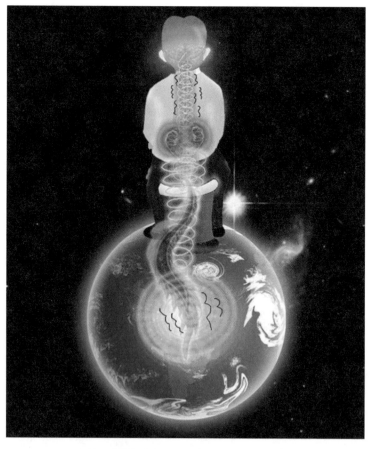

Fig. 2.32. Wagging the Dragon's Tail

After doing some or all of these exercises, notice what feels different to you in terms of your energy, body, emotions, and the quality of your thoughts.

Other Exercises for Awakening the Core Link

It is important to highlight that the exercises shown in this book are just examples. The Universal Healing Tao system offers a wealth of practices and now that you understand the concepts of Flow, you can apply them to any and all of the practices. For example, breath work activates the respiratory and cardio pumps. Any of the exercises that pump the legs or tilt and tuck the pelvis will encourage more flow in the sacral pump. Exercises that move the neck will open the flow of the cranial pump.

In addition to the individual exercises mentioned here, Tai Chi practice is especially good for awakening the cranial and sacral pumps and all the pumps in between. In Tai Chi, each movement comes from the feet, the motion of the sacrum, and lower tan tien. As the foot steps down on the earth, the pressure transfers up the legs to the pelvis and through the spine. This rippling of the spine activates the cranial and sacral pumps and increases the flow of cerebrospinal fluid throughout the entire system. Earlier, we learned that the flow of CSF is critical for our health and well-being because of its role in nourishing the brain and protecting the immune system. This information offers a physiological explanation for many of the great health benefits attributed to the ancient art of Tai Chi.

In addition to the four major pumps we have explored in this chapter, there are many more pumps in the body, each helping to move fluids and energy throughout the entire system. These other pumps can be activated with various Chi Kung exercises. For example, many of the Tan Tien Chi Kung exercises twist the spine to open other important pumps at C7 and T11. As you practice, begin to notice which pumps are activated by each exercise. The more that you understand their purpose, the more effective they will become.

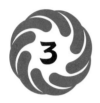

Building Awareness and Appreciation

Once you've awakened the four major pumps in the three tan tiens, you can work to increase your awareness and appreciation of the Flow they create.

BUILDING AWARENESS
Listening for Flow in the Body

Building awareness is important not only for your physical health, but for your spiritual growth as well. Lao Tzu teaches us that knowing others is intelligence, but knowing yourself is true wisdom.[1]

Each of the following exercises builds your capacity to notice physical flow and hones your skill in tracking it.

 ## Following the Breath

One easy way to bring your awareness to the body and its natural rhythms is to tune in to your breath. This exercise (and the ones that follow) brings your awareness to the four characteristics of Flow that we introduced earlier: tempo (how fast or slow you are breathing), magnitude (how shallow or deep), balance (how equal your inhalations and exhalations), and quality (how you would describe your breath).

The exercise can be done standing, sitting, or lying down.

1. Close your eyes. Place one hand gently on your chest and the other hand on your belly (see fig. 3.1 on page 66). Bring your awareness to your breath and simply breathe normally.
2. Tune in to your inhalations and exhalations.
3. Become aware of the tempo of your breath and observe how the speed changes as you relax.
4. Notice the depth and volume of your inhalations and exhalations; notice how these features change as your breath becomes fuller.
5. Compare your inhalation to your exhalation. It may be shorter or longer; it may be easier or more difficult.
6. Describe the quality of your breath. Sense whether it feels relatively rushed, choppy, strained, or steady, even, and full. Allow yourself to notice these characteristics of your breath without judgment.
7. Whatever you observe, just relax and feel the flow of your breath moving throughout your body.
8. Observe whether the hand at your chest moves with your inhalation and exhalation. Do the same with the hand on your belly.
9. Notice where your breath seems to move easily and also any areas where it may flow less freely.
10. Invite any areas of constriction to soften and the breath to move into those regions.
11. As you become more mindful of your breath, allow it to deepen and become slower, smoother, and more even. As you breathe more fully and deeply, you naturally become more relaxed.
12. Connect the in-breath with the out-breath until you're breathing is one continuous circuit, as if a wave is ebbing and flowing throughout your whole body.

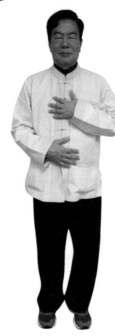

Fig. 3.1. Following the Breath

During this exercise, you may become aware that your heart rate slows, your emotions calm, and your mind clears and settles. The gentle yet powerful flow of breath encourages the movement of energy throughout your entire system.

By building awareness of your breath, you can become conscious of the flow of air through your system, which in turn helps you track your energy flow. Once you are aware of Flow in any form, you can use the power of intention along with Chi Kung exercises to enhance and optimize it.

Listening to the Heart Flow

In this exercise, you will improve your ability to listen to the flow of the heart. True listening is not just noticing, but entails being completely present with what you are experiencing.

1. Sit or lie comfortably.
2. Bring your hands to your heart and your attention to your heartbeat (fig. 3.2). Notice the tempo of your heartbeat. The rate might

be fast like a racehorse, slow like a turtle floating in a calm and sheltered cove, or somewhere in between.

3. Place your awareness on the strength and power (or magnitude) of the beat.

4. Check in to see how balanced the beat feels. It might feel hollow and tentative. It might be full and robust. Just notice how it feels to you.

5. Sense the beating of the heart and the movement of blood that is pumping throughout your entire body.

6. Rest in that flow for a while.

7. Now, widen your perception of your heart to more than its rhythm. Pay attention to how it feels more generally. Find words to describe the quality of your whole heart field in this moment. For example, some hearts feel tired from carrying heavy burdens and seem to be looking for rest. Other hearts feel light and buoyant, ready to enjoy and explore. Listen for the message that your heart is telling you.

8. There are no right or wrong answers; just allow yourself to become aware of and connected to your heart in a new and deeper way.

9. Now let that go and return to deep and even natural breathing.

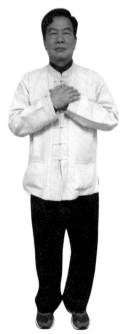

Fig. 3.2. Listening to the Heart Flow

Tuning In to Specific Flows

Once you have learned to recognize Flow in your body, you can tune in to specific aspects of it. Our bodies have many different rhythms. Like a radio, we "broadcast" several different programs at a time (fig. 3.3). Just as we scan the airwaves with a radio dial and tune in to the program we want to receive, we can similarly scan our bodies and tune in to the particular rhythm we want to work with. The Cranial Wave, for example, is the flow that connects the cranium with the sacrum. A complete cycle of this wave up and down the spine occurs roughly 8–14 times per minute. If you are sensing something moving at that tempo, you have likely tuned in to the Cranial Wave. If you notice something moving significantly faster or slower than that, you are probably tapping into a different "program"— just relax and continue to listen for a rhythm that takes about three seconds to travel along the spine in one direction and three seconds to return.

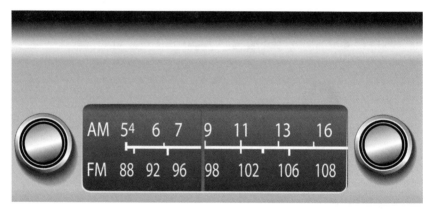

Fig. 3.3. Tuning in to the Flow

 Connecting to the Core Link

Feeling the Cranial Wave

Remember that the sacrum and occiput are paired bones, connected by the dura mater, the tube that protects the spinal cord. The dural tube reaches all the way from the occiput down to S2, the second

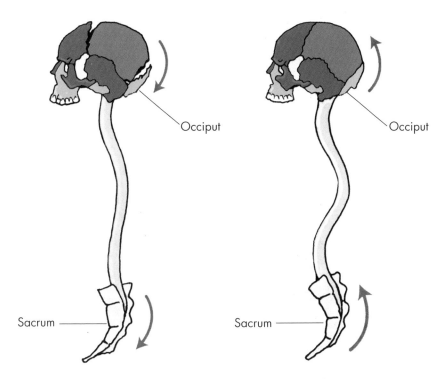

Fig. 3.4. Sacrum and occiput
in synchrony, inhalation

Fig. 3.5. Sacrum and occiput
in synchrony, exhalation

sacral segment. Because of this elastic connection, the two bones move together. On inhalation, they both move down (inferior) and the bottom aspect of each bone moves slightly forward (anterior) (fig. 3.4). On exhalation, they both move up (superior) and the bottom aspect of each bone moves slightly posterior (fig. 3.5).

1. Stand with your feet shoulder-width apart and knees bent slightly.
2. Place one hand on your occiput at the base of the skull and the other hand on your sacrum (see fig. 3.6 on page 70). Feel the similarity in the curves between the two bones.
3. Now sense the connection between your hands. Feel the spine, the spinal cord, and the dura that connects the bones.
4. Sense into this vertical core and bring your awareness to any

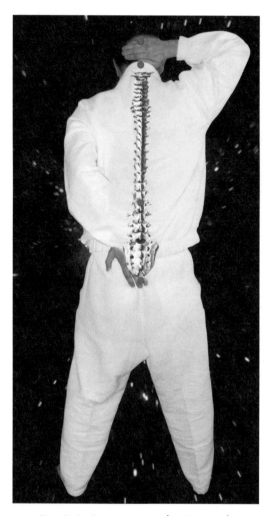

Fig. 3.6. Connecting to the Core Link

rhythms you find moving there. Feel how the two bones have similar patterns of motion—as the sacrum tucks, the head moves backward slightly.

5. You may observe a subtle sense of movement flowing from your tailbone up through your spine and neck to your cranium and back down again. It may feel like heat or tingling in a particular area, or along the whole spine. It may flow like a wave or move bit by bit. If this movement takes about 3 seconds to ascend and 3 seconds

to descend, then you are sensing the tempo and movement of the Cranial Wave.

6. Notice the magnitude of the wave-like movement. Pay attention to whether this feels like a kiddie-pool wave, a tsunami, or something in between.

7. Consider the balance of the wave by paying attention to whether the flow up the spine seems balanced with the downward movement. Notice if the flow in one direction feels stronger, smoother, or easier than in the other direction.

8. And lastly, observe the overall quality of the Flow—not of the bones. Perhaps the movement feels heavy and sluggish or buoyant and exuberant. Find the words that best describe your Flow in this moment.

When you first begin to build awareness, it may be challenging to find words that describe what you are sensing. Yet part of increasing your awareness is being able to articulate what you notice: the more that you are able to name the nuances, the greater your ability to notice subtle variations. Improving the wiring in one area helps to improve the wiring in the other.

Note: The healthy "normal" movement of the sacrum and occiput is to dance together in synchrony. If you notice a pattern of opposite movement or a lag between their movements, just gently invite them to synchronize. Over time, the Taoist practices will foster improved communication between these two poles, which will help them connect more easily and deeply.

During Spinal Cord Breathing, we intentionally move the sacrum and occiput in opposite directions to stimulate the pumps and increase their activity. Likewise in Tai Chi and Chi Kung, it is common to create a slight oppositional movement that enlivens the flow of chi when we gently tuck both the pelvis and the chin, while moving the crown to the sky and gently elongating the neck. In these cases, when we finish practicing, synchronized movement returns naturally.

Connecting the Pumps

This exercise helps you expand your awareness further by sensing all of the pumps interacting at once. Start by rotating your awareness through each of the pumps; over time, you will begin to feel them all at once.

1. Place your hands wherever they are comfortable and close your eyes, bringing your awareness inside.
2. Tune in to your breath and the flow of the air through your system (figs. 3.7 and 3.8).

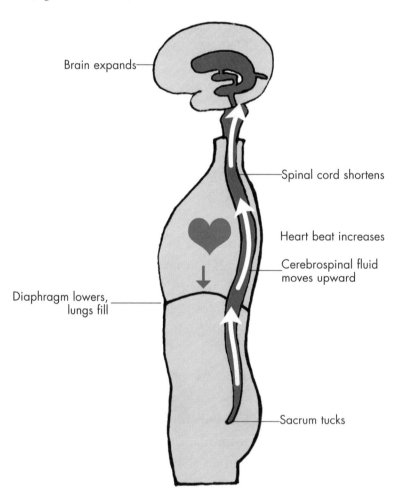

Brain expands

Spinal cord shortens

Heart beat increases

Cerebrospinal fluid
moves upward

Diaphragm lowers,
lungs fill

Sacrum tucks

Fig. 3.7. The pumps during inhalation

3. Sense your heart beat and the pumping of blood through your whole body.
4. Open your awareness to your sacrum and occiput. Feel CSF moving through the brain and spinal cord like a tide.
5. Sense the rhythm of the tide drawing in and expanding out.
6. Feel yourself as a three-dimensional fluid body moving with these tides. Let go of any need to control the tide, simply relax into it.
7. Allow the body's inner wisdom and capacity for healing to harmonize and realign whatever is necessary to optimize your systems.

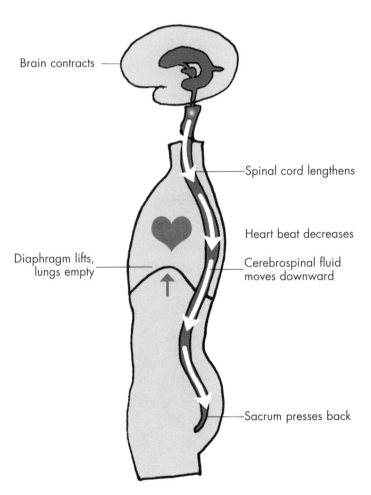

Fig. 3.8. The pumps during exhalation

Noticing Signs of Improved Flow

As physical flow increases, you may notice the following common shifts:

- Changes in breath rate, heart rate, temperature sensations (of heat or coolness), and/or skin color changes
- A sense of relaxation, softening, opening, spreading, and/or expansion
- Energy flow changes, pulsing sensations, meridian flow shifts, feeling energized as well as relaxed
- Noises—bubbling, gas, gurgling, fluid releases
- Micro movements, twitches, quivering, shaking, or trembling
- Coughing, yawning, sighing
- Emotional release—crying, laughing, shouting, groaning, joyfulness

APPRECIATING THE FLOW

Now that we have awakened and brought our awareness to the Flow through each of the major pumps, we begin to appreciate that Flow more deeply. As in daily life, appreciation enhances our emotional satisfaction and well-being. It also helps us absorb and integrate the benefits of Flow into our lives.

Recent research in the field of positive psychology provides scientific support for the idea that appreciation produces significant and long-lasting health benefits (fig. 3.9). In one study of people suffering from various neuromuscular diseases, those who were encouraged to spend time in appreciation by writing gratitude journals reported getting more sleep, spending less time awake before falling asleep, and feeling more refreshed in the morning.[2]

Researchers at the University of Connecticut found that gratitude can also have a protective effect against heart attacks. In the study, researchers found that patients who focused on the positive aspects of what they had learned after the heart attack and reported appreciation for how their life changed had a lower risk of subsequent heart attacks.[3]

Other studies show that gratitude corresponds with longer life as well as lower levels of depression and other diseases. Additional research has found that people who practice mindful appreciation experience greater emotional resilience and also:

- Take better care of themselves physically and mentally
- Engage in more regular exercise
- Eat a healthier diet
- Have improved mental alertness
- Cope better with stress
- Experience fewer physical problems
- Have stronger immune systems

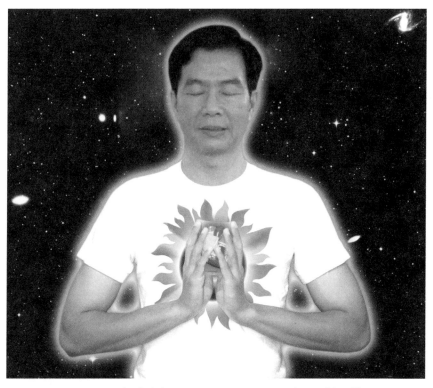

Fig. 3.9. The link between appreciation and good health

Focusing Appreciation with the Inner Smile

The Inner Smile is one of the simplest, yet most profound, Chi Kung practices. In the exercises below, you can use the Inner Smile to focus your appreciation on the four major pumps of your body as well as on your capacity to sustain good flow.

 Appreciating the Pumps

In this exercise, you'll use the Inner Smile meditation to help you maintain and sustain your physical flow.

1. Bring your awareness to your sacrum and to the cranial pump at the base of your skull (the occiput). Feel their connection and the cerebrospinal fluid flowing easily from one to the other along the spinal cord. Smile into the sacrum and occiput and appreciate their strength, stability, and power (fig. 3.10).

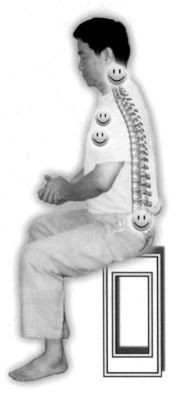

Fig. 3.10. Appreciating our pumps

2. Bring your awareness into your lungs and heart. Sense the respiratory pump oxygenating your blood and the cardiac pump circulating that blood in your whole body. Smile into your heart and lungs.

3. As you inhale smiling energy, imagine an ocean wave gathering and storing up power and potency. As you exhale, feel that wave flowing outward bringing oxygen, blood, and cerebrospinal fluid to your entire body.

4. Notice how the Inner Smile enhances the Flow, making it more fluid, natural, and effortless.

Sustaining the Flow

More generally, we can use the Inner Smile to help us sustain the Flow of our overall health.

1. Find a comfortable position either sitting or lying.

2. Recall a time when you sensed good physical flow. Perhaps it was a time when you felt physically fit and healthy. It might be a time when you achieved a challenging physical goal or a day when everything went right while playing sports. It could be a treasured memory of enjoying a hike. It might be recent or it might be long ago.

3. Bring this time to mind and feel how it felt in your body to have things working well.

4. If it has been so long since you felt physical flow that you cannot remember it clearly, then simply imagine what it would feel like to have all of the internal systems of your body working smoothly and effortlessly.

5. Sense the pumps open and activated, moving all fluids freely and easily.

6. Feel your body strong and supple, moving gracefully and powerfully.

7. As you remember or imagine what that felt like, smile. Smile with the joy of feeling that healthy and vital (figs. 3.11 and 3.12 on page 78).

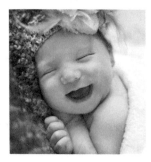

Fig. 3.11. Being awake, aware, and appreciative sustains the Flow.

8. Relax and breathe deeply. Let your Inner Smile deepen. Send appreciation and gratitude to all of the many parts of your body that are working together, each one doing its job well.

9. As you rest in appreciation, feel your physical flow become more tangible, more palpable, and more manifest. The more that you feel in Flow, the more that you will be in Flow.

10. Spending a few moments each day with the Inner Smile will encourage this felt sense of Flow and help to sustain it.

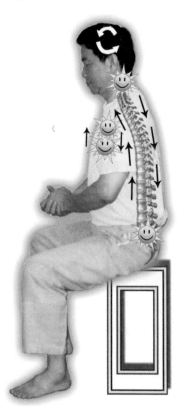

Fig. 3.12. Becoming aware and appreciating the pumps

PART TWO

Emotional and Mental Flows

In the preceding chapters we have seen how Flow contributes to physical health and vitality. In the next section, we will look at how Flow can bring greater harmony into our lives and assist with our emotional and mental well-being.

Balancing Flow in these areas is important because when we experience too little movement in our emotions and thoughts, we can feel stuck, uncreative, unproductive, or helpless. When there is too much movement, we may feel flighty, volatile, unstable, or unable to focus or concentrate. All too often, however, we either ignore our mental/emotional flow or feel powerless to change it. The good news is that once we understand how these flows work, we can harmonize our emotions and thoughts with simple, yet effective practices.

In part 2, we will begin by looking at the importance of building awareness of our emotional flow. We will then explore recent research that explores the connection between our head, heart, and gut brains, and how these three intelligences communicate. Throughout, we will highlight the similarities between Tai Chi and craniosacral principles and how they can be applied to increasing our emotional and mental fluidity. To do this, we will develop our skills in Listening, Following, and Unwinding, and combine them with Universal Healing Tao practices to help bring mindful balance to our emotional and mental flows.

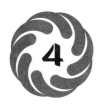

Everything Is Connected to the Flow

While most of us appreciate our good feelings, we often try to push away the negative ones, hoping to feel good all of the time. However, even unpleasant feelings are part of our dynamic Flow and can help us to increase our health and vitality.

ACCESSING THE FULL SPECTRUM OF OUR EMOTIONS

Our thoughts and emotions are powerful and can lead to strong—and sometimes uncomfortable—sensations. In our ongoing natural attempts to move away from pain and toward comfort, our subconscious will label some thoughts or emotions as "bad." As a result, we shy away from them and, over time, become more and more reluctant to experience them.

However, we truly limit ourselves when we refuse to experience some of our emotions. It is like limiting our ability to see certain parts of the visual spectrum: some "colors" become unavailable to us. Although we might prefer some colors to others, being able to see the entire spectrum adds vibrancy to our lives (see fig. 4.1 on page 82). If we saw only one or two colors, we wouldn't be able to experience life in the same way.

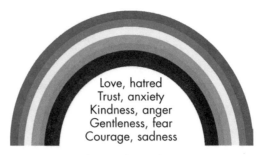

Love, hatred
Trust, anxiety
Kindness, anger
Gentleness, fear
Courage, sadness

Fig. 4.1. The rainbow of our emotions

Sometimes the discomfort of challenging emotions causes us to stuff them deep down inside and try to lock them away. Because there is no Flow, these emotions accumulate and build up pressure. Eventually, they may burst out despite our best efforts. For some people, alternating between no emotional flow and excessive emotional flow seems normal: Chi Kung practices aim to smooth out these flows so that we can experience all of our emotions fully, as well as express them skillfully and authentically.

We can relate these ideas to the Tai Chi form. We may notice that we move more easily in one direction than another. Perhaps we have an old injury on one side that causes us discomfort to the point that we dislike moving in that direction. Over time, if we avoid moving toward that side, we will lose more and more mobility. A dedicated Tai Chi practitioner will use the form to observe areas of tension and restriction. Each day, he will go up to the point of discomfort without forcing his body to go further and relax there, appreciating what his body is able to do. As the tension releases, he may be able to go a little bit further, a little deeper. Over time, his range of motion and capability will increase until he is able to flow easily in all directions. We can use this same method to release physical, emotional, and mental restrictions.

Appreciating the Gift of our Emotions

You may be thinking that experiencing positive emotions such as joy, kindness, and courage is well and good, but that you do not particularly want to experience impatience, anger, or sadness. It is easy for us to understand the benefits of our positive emotions because they feel good, but it can be more difficult for us to acknowledge the gifts that our challenging emotions bring as well. Often, it is the discomfort of negative emotions that awakens us to their presence and increases our awareness of what needs our attention. And it is that same discomfort that creates motivation for us to move mindfully toward harmony and balance. The more discomfort, the more we are motivated to do something about it. Emotions provide us with valuable feedback and guidance; even the uncomfortable ones. It is only when our emotions get stuck or we ignore them that they create problems. Rather than avoiding negative emotions, our focus should be on encouraging optimal Flow so that they arise, present their gifts, and then dissipate in a healthy way.

In Taoism and Chinese medicine, we use the framework of the five elements and their associated emotions, both positive and negative (fig. 4.2). A chart of the five elements and their gifts appears on page 84. The more

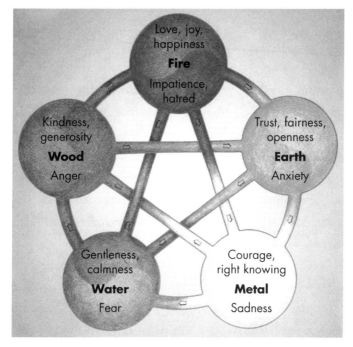

Fig. 4.2. The five elements and their related emotions

that we recognize the gifts inherent in challenging emotions, the more willing we will be to experience, accept, and benefit from what they offer.

THE GIFTS OF CHALLENGING EMOTIONS

ELEMENT	POSITIVE EMOTIONS	CHALLENGING EMOTIONS AND THEIR GIFTS
Fire	Love, joy, happiness	Impatience/hatred: reveals the ways in which we create separation from others and invites us to connect with them.
Earth	Trust, fairness, openness	Anxiety: encourages us toward comfort and stability.
Metal	Courage, right-knowing	Sadness: sensitizes us to pain and loss and moves us toward clarity and connection with spirit.
Water	Gentleness, calmness	Fear: causes us to pay attention to our safety, protection, and self-care.
Wood	Kindness, generosity	Anger: motivates us to change and grow.

EMOTIONAL INTELLIGENCE

Since the groundbreaking work on emotional intelligence done by psychologists Peter Salovey and John Mayer and popularized by Daniel Goleman in the 1990s, Western society has begun to acknowledge the important influence of emotional intelligence on both our well-being and on our ability to navigate life successfully (fig. 4.3).[1] The fundamental building blocks of our emotional intelligence are our capacities for self-awareness, self-management, social awareness, and relationship management.

- **Self-awareness** is our ability to access and name our experiences, including our feelings, thoughts, wants, intentions, and body sensations. Self-awareness allows us to observe our thoughts, feelings, and behaviors in the moment as we participate in life.

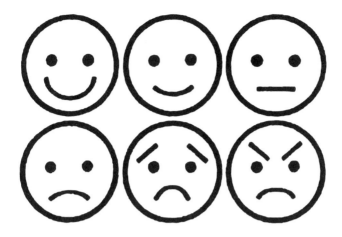

Fig. 4.3. Emotional intelligence

- **Self-management** or self-soothing is our ability to experience any discomfort and manage it in ways that help us regain our equilibrium.
- **Social awareness** or empathy is our ability to identify and understand other people's wants, needs, and concerns.
- **Relationship management** is our ability to develop and maintain good relationships, communicate clearly, as well as inspire and influence others.

Increasing Emotional Intelligence

Taoism offers us the opportunity to use meditation and physical exercises to build our self-awareness. The Universal Healing Tao formulas provide processes for skillful self-management so that we can return to harmony once we notice our own imbalances. The spiritual aspects and connection with Oneness that are part of the practices (which we will explore more deeply later in the book) build and develop our capacity for social awareness and responsible relationship management.

Goleman quotes Aristotle at the beginning of *Emotional Intelligence*: "Anyone can become angry—that is easy. But to be angry with the right person, to the right degree, at the right time, for the right purpose, and in the right way—this is not easy."[2] Additionally, to be able to release that anger and reharmonize ourselves is another level of refinement. Taoist Chi Kung helps us build the skills that enable us to be truly emotionally intelligent.

Connecting Our Sensing, Feeling, and Thinking

In Eastern philosophies, the Heart (that which feels) and Mind (that which perceives and thinks) are so closely related as to be virtually inseparable. Translators of the ancient texts often refer to the combined concept as the Heart/Mind.

In the West, the Cartesian approach—a strong influence in philosophy since the 1600s—promoted the idea of separation between sensing, feeling, and rational thinking. More recently, however, scientific studies have revealed the fundamental interconnections between thinking and feeling.

Cognitive psychology suggests that we receive information about the world around us through our sense organs and use our thoughts (our perceptions, beliefs, and attitudes) to interpret that information. Both the sensory data and our thoughts about it are required to bring meaning to our lives. Emotional intelligence studies suggest that we take in information through three filters: our physical sensations, our emotional responses, and our mental perceptions. Information is available from all three channels, but each individual relies on the different channels to a different extent.

Current neuroscience suggests that simply *thinking about* ideas or events activates the sympathetic nervous system and emotions in the same ways that experiencing those things would.[3] If we recall a relaxing vacation, for instance, we feel peaceful and our nervous system actually calms (fig. 4.4).

Emotions do not "get in the way" of rational thinking; emotions are essential to rationality. Studies on decision making show that purely rational decisions are not optimal: emotions are vital for good

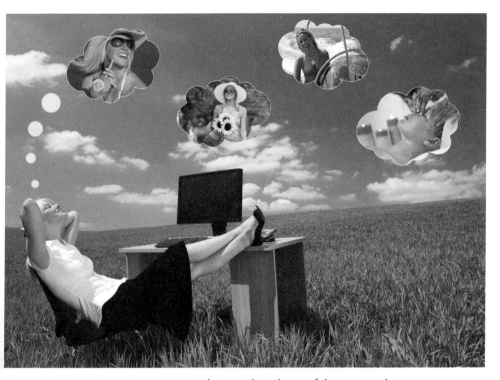

Fig. 4.4. We respond to our thoughts as if they are real.

decision making and intelligent choices. The orbitofrontal cortex of the brain connects feelings to conscious thought. People with brain damage in this area cannot integrate their emotional and cognitive systems. In other words, they are unable to respond emotionally to the content of their thoughts and therefore are not able to make appropriate judgments or plans because they are missing critical input from their internal stimuli. They have tremendous difficulty making decisions and can no longer function effectively, even though their mental abilities are considered to be normal. These patients demonstrate that when we don't know how we feel about something, we lose access to the power of our subconscious thinking. We literally do not know what to think.

External stimuli from our senses and internal stimuli from our emotions combine to influence our decisions and actions. Consciousness

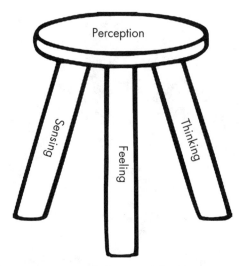

Fig. 4.5. How sensing, feeling, and thinking are connected

(awareness of inner states) evolved because it allows us to use our emotions to evaluate external information (fig. 4.5). This process of evaluation is usually significantly faster than our cognitive assessment.

Healing on Multiple Levels

Because of these deep connections, lack of Flow on one level affects Flow on other levels. For example, poor flow in our mental or emotional bodies often shows up as tension in or issues with our physical body: emotional experiences, thoughts, and memories not only affect us in the moment but are also stored in the body. The good news about these connections is that any work that balances one level will improve balance on the others.

As bodyworkers and people who receive transformational bodywork know, when physical tension is released, emotions, thoughts, or memories may surface to be released as well. It is also true that emotional or psychological healing often leads to improvements in long-standing physical conditions. Of course this makes sense because we are not just a collection of parts; all of our parts work together and form an integrated and connected whole.

HEAD BRAIN, HEART BRAIN, AND GUT BRAIN

Most people in the West believe that we only have one brain; the one in our heads. However, medical research is coming to understand what Taoists have known for millennia, that we have at least three brains. These three brains—the head brain, heart brain, and gut brain— correlate with the three tan tiens (fig. 4.6).

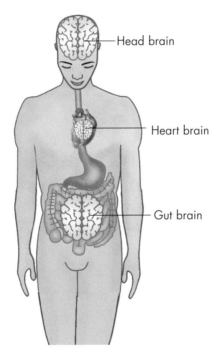

Fig. 4.6. Brains in our tan tiens

Understanding the Heart Brain

More than just a pump, the heart is also a sensory organ and a sophis-ticated center for receiving and processing information. The nervous system within the heart—the heart brain—enables it to sense, learn, remember, and make functional decisions independent of the head brain.

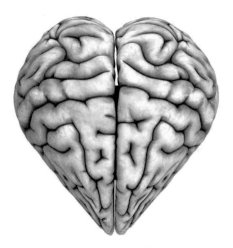

Fig. 4.7. Heart brain

The heart brain is in constant communication with the head brain and the rest of the body, influencing function, information processing, perceptions, emotions, and health. The heart communicates neurologically (through transmissions of nerve impulses); biochemically (through hormones and neurotransmitters); biophysically (through pressure waves); and energetically (through electromagnetic field interactions).

Historically, Western scientists have focused primarily on the heart's responses to the head brain's commands, believing that the head brain was in charge of running the body's systems. However, technological advances now allow us to understand more about head/heart communication. More recent data shows that communication between the heart and head is a dynamic, ongoing dialogue, with each organ continuously influencing the other's functions.

The heart has its own nervous system, which contains approximately forty thousand neurons. These neurons detect hormones and neurochemicals and sense heart rate and pressure information. Two-way communication between the cognitive and emotional systems is hardwired into the brain; the actual number of neural connections going from the emotional centers to the cognitive centers is greater than the number going the other way.

Although Western medicine has viewed emotions as mental expressions generated by the head brain, recent studies show that neurological and hormonal signals from many organs, including the heart, influence perceptual and emotional processing in the head brain. Our physical, emotional, and mental health has been linked to the production and balance of our neurochemicals. In the past, it was assumed that the head brain was the predominant producer of these key substances. However, the head does not have a monopoly on their production. The heart also produces neurotransmitters critical for our core functioning. For example, the heart creates the neurohormone, atrial natriuretic factor (ANF), which communicates with the brain and immune system. It influences our blood vessels, kidneys, adrenal glands, thalamus, hypothalamus, pineal, and pituitary glands, as well as several regulatory regions in the brain.

The heart also secretes oxytocin, which is involved in a host of social activities including our levels of tolerance, complex sexual and maternal behaviors, the learning of social cues, and the establishment of pair bonding. Concentrations of oxytocin in the heart are as high as those found in the brain. This may be why the heart has been linked to our social interactions in many cultures throughout our history.

It is clear that what goes on in the heart affects our other systems. For example, when we are in love, our hearts secrete oxytocin. If you have ever talked with someone who is in love, it is easy to notice how strongly emotions influence their thinking and behavior. Thanks to science and technology, we now understand the physiological basis for this connection.

Emotions and the Heart Brain

According to the HeartMath Institute, strong emotions easily draw our attention and influence our thoughts. However, thoughts do not so easily displace emotions from our conscious mind. Previous emotional experiences are powerful influencers of our future attitudes, reactions, and behaviors.[4]

Because emotions have such a potent influence on our mental body, addressing issues at the emotional level can be effective in changing cognitive patterns and processes. Increasing harmony in the emotional system can often bring the mind into greater harmony as well.

Our emotional state is communicated throughout the body via the magnitude, pattern, and tempo of the heartbeat. As we experience different emotions, our heartbeat changes significantly. Negative emotions, such as anger or frustration, are associated with erratic, disorganized patterns in the heart's rhythms (fig. 4.8). These are stressful for the nervous system and consume more energy.

Heart rhythms also affect our perceptive and cognitive capacities. A heart experiencing stress transmits disorganized signals to the brain, reducing our ability to focus, remember, learn, solve problems, and think clearly. Changes in the heartbeat also alter the flow of oxygen and nutrients throughout the body, which is one reason why our emotional state has such a strong overall effect on our health.

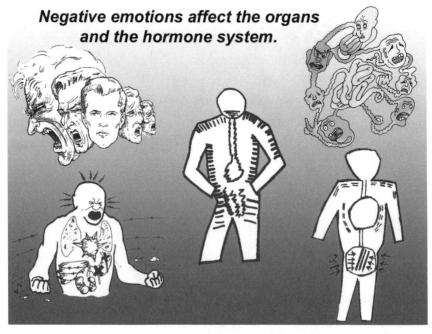

Fig. 4.8. Emotions influence the physical body.

In contrast, positive emotions, such as love or appreciation, correlate with more consistent organized patterns in the heart's rhythmic activity and in the structure of the electromagnetic field radiated by the heart. As the heart's electromagnetic field becomes more ordered, physical benefits include increased efficiency and harmony in the nervous, cardiovascular, hormonal, and immune systems, as well as reduced stress. The mental and emotional benefits of greater organization include reduced internal mental chatter, improved mental clarity and cognitive performance, greater emotional stability, and more accurate intuition.

Respecting our Gut Brain

In addition to a head brain and heart brain, we also have a gut brain—our enteric nervous system (ENS) (fig. 4.9). Author Michael Gershon finds that the West has been aware of the second brain for the last century.[5] Gershon reports that the enteric nervous system has over 100

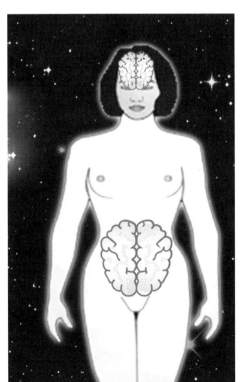

Fig. 4.9. Gut brain

million neurons embedded in it, which is more than the spinal cord or peripheral nervous system. This gut brain has its own sensory systems and reflexes as well as the capacity to feel, learn, and remember. It does so differently than the head brain, and in ways that the head brain cannot consciously access.

The ENS can operate without input from the head brain, making and executing its own decisions. Most of the chemicals that influence the head brain are also present in the gut. The ENS produces and uses more than thirty neurotransmitters including serotonin, glutamate, dopamine, acetylcholine, and norepinephrine. Over 90 percent of the body's serotonin and 50 percent of the body's dopamine are found in the gut. The gut also functions as our body's anxiety and pain reliever, producing benzodiazepines that are similar to drugs like Valium and Xanax. Gastrointestinal difficulties affect our mood and cognition while stress and emotional challenges can derail our digestion. Although we may not want to acknowledge it, many of our emotional responses, moods, and feelings of well-being are influenced by our gut.

Communication between the Gut Brain and the Head Brain

Communication between the gut and head brains is important for our health and survival. The head brain communicates with the gut brain by using command neurons to carry messages up and down the system. Command neurons control the pattern of activity in the gut, while the vagus nerve alters the volume by changing its rates of firing. During stressful situations, the head signals the gut to secrete histamine, prostaglandin, and other substances that produce inflammation. However, these chemicals may also cause diarrhea and cramping. During periods of prolonged stress, the chronic inflammation and intestinal distress negatively affect our health, mood, and vitality. Common issues such as anxiety, depression, irritable bowel syndrome, ulcers, and Parkinson's disease cause symptoms in both the head and gut brains.

The gut can upset the brain just as the brain upsets the gut. Between

80 to 90 percent of the nerve fibers of the vagus nerve are dedicated to sending sensory data from our organs to the brain. However, stress can create muscular contractions that turn into knots. These knots may press against the nerves and the lumbar/sacral plexus, negatively impacting the flow of important messages from the viscera to the brain and vice versa.

Knots are surface blockages that can entangle with the fascia and lymph. Tangles occur more deeply than knots and involve the larger structures of nerves, lymph, tendons, muscles, arteries, veins, and fascia, as well as the organ systems and their energies. When emotional tensions are stored in the gut, they can lead to muscular contractions in the back, legs, and psoas muscles. Over time, the tightness may irritate the nerves elsewhere, causing pain. This is why pressing on the abdomen may trigger pain in other areas. Freeing knots and tangles allows the blood, chi, emotions, and thoughts to flow freely. We can see that the health of the gut brain plays an important role in our physical, emotional, and mental lives.

The Gut Brain Is the Lower Tan Tien

Taoism has acknowledged the importance of the gut brain or lower tan tien for over five thousand years. In Taoism, the lower tan tien is seen as a place to unify body, mind, and spirit; problems in this area can affect our overall energy. The small intestine, for example, is in charge of digesting emotions as well as food. Tension in this organ can be related to undigested negative emotions—especially hatred and impatience.

Beyond the small intestine, we can correlate imbalances in particular emotions with tightness and pain in certain regions. For example, anger affects the upper right side near the liver; worry causes tension in the upper left side near the spleen. Anxiety is near the top and sadness affects both lower lateral sides. Fear causes reactions in the deep lower areas. When we open and release the gut, we harmonize our emotions and improve our cognition. We also open our consciousness to the wisdom and knowingness found in the lower tan tien.

THE RELATIONSHIP OF
ELEMENTS, ORGANS, AND EMOTIONS

ELEMENT	ORGANS	CHALLENGING EMOTIONS
Fire	Heart/Small Intestine	Impatience/hatred
Earth	Stomach/Spleen/Pancreas	Anxiety
Metal	Lungs/Large Intestine	Sadness
Water	Kidneys/Bladder	Fear
Wood	Liver/Gall Bladder	Anger

The table above shows the relationships between the five elements and the organs, and the challenging emotions associated with them. The next figure shows the location of those organs in the body (fig. 4.10), and the following figure shows how we may experience the challenging emotions in those organs (fig. 4.11).

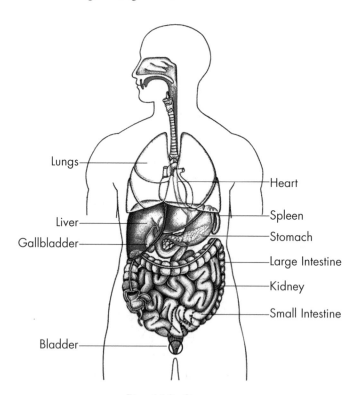

Fig. 4.10. Organs

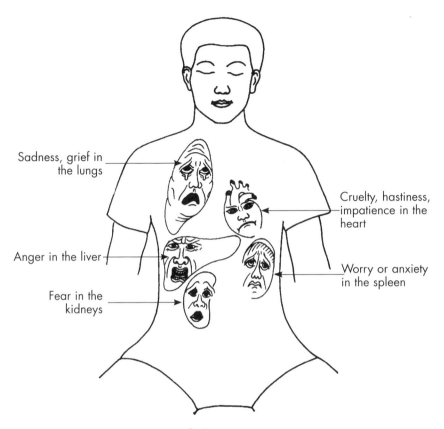

Sadness, grief in
the lungs

Cruelty, hastiness,
impatience in the
heart

Anger in the liver

Worry or anxiety
in the spleen

Fear in the
kidneys

Fig. 4.11. We feel emotions in our organs.

Using Leverage to Create Flow in Many Dimensions of Being

The deep, multilayered interconnections among our physical, emotional, and mental bodies mean that we have three powerful levers we can use on our journey toward greater Flow and harmony. In some situations, it is possible to work directly with the area in which we are experiencing difficulties. If we have a physical issue, we can work on it with physical means. However, sometimes the issues are deeper, more complex, or more challenging and may be less responsive to direct methods. In such cases, it can be helpful to use one of the other levers to create an opening for shifts. Because our physical, emotional, and

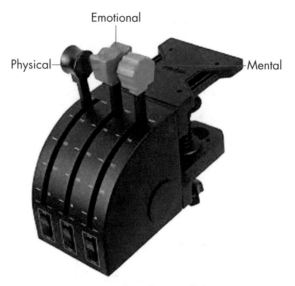

Fig. 4.12. Three levels of change

mental bodies are related, if we change one, the others must change as well (fig. 4.12).

For example, we may know that our emotions or thoughts are stuck in certain holding patterns, but we may not know how to increase fluidity and create change in such intangible areas. In this case, releasing tension, increasing flexibility, and reharmonizing the physical body can assist the emotional and mental bodies in coming into better balance as well. In the next chapters, we will practice working with all three levers to build better Flow throughout our entire being.

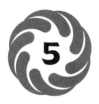

Balancing Emotional and Mental Flows

After becoming familiar with the physical flows of the Core Link, the next step in working with Flow is to recognize the mental and emotional energies moving through us. Both craniosacral workers and Tai Chi practitioners use similar principles in addressing these less tangible aspects of Flow.

CRANIOSACRAL METHODS OF APPRECIATING MENTAL AND EMOTIONAL FLOWS

In Craniosacral Work, practitioners learn to address emotional and mental flows with a series of practices referred to as *listening, following,* and *unwinding.*

Listening with the Heart

In Craniosacral Work, *listening* has a particular meaning. It means being able to observe what *is* without judgment. When we listen in this way, we listen with our hands, our chi, and our presence, not just with our head or ears.

Most importantly, however, we also listen with our heart (fig. 5.1). About 400 AD, Saint Benedict made a point of emphasizing that the foundation for the organization he was creating would be *asculta*. Asculta means listening, but a special kind of listening—listening with the heart; it is a different experience, powerful and deeply healing.

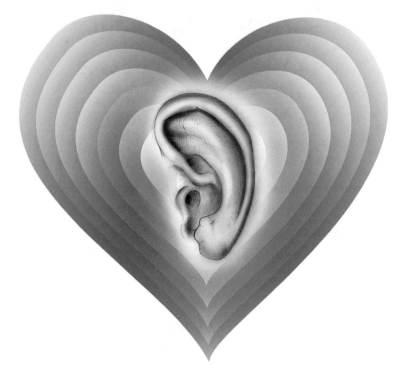

Fig. 5.1. Listening with the heart

To understand the power of listening with the heart, try listening to some music with your ears (just hearing the sounds), or with your head (thinking about the composition or the execution). Then listen to the same piece with your heart. Notice the difference.

You might also apply this to listening to a colleague telling you about an issue at work. Consider whether your response would be different if you also listened with your heart rather than just with your head. What difference would that make to your colleague and the way he or she then chooses to handle the situation?

Following the Flow

Following means that we are so connected with the structure or energy channel we are touching that we can stay with it as it moves. When we are following, we are in perfect synchrony: we do not judge, change, exaggerate, or resist the movement. As we work with following, it is helpful to know a little more about direction of movement.

When we tuned in to the Cranial Wave in chapter 3, we noticed that there was a sense of movement. In which direction was it going? Rather than anatomical or geographical references, craniosacral practitioners use the terms "direction of ease" and "direction of discomfort" to describe the vector of movement.

Movement in the direction of ease is characterized by sensations of fluidity, lightness, buoyancy, pleasure, and joy. People are usually comfortable with movement in this direction. When movement is in the direction of discomfort, on the other hand, we may experience any or all of the following:

- Physical discomfort, numbness, or pain
- Changes in speed and quality of movement—dragging, freezing, resistance, spasms, roughness, ratcheting, sluggishness, or congestion
- Increased tension, density, or heaviness
- Lack of vitality or sparkle
- Emotional discomfort: vulnerability, sadness, safety issues, checking out, leaving the body, fear, anxiety, wanting to stop or leave
- Disturbing images or pictures

When we follow, we stay with the structure until it reaches its limit of movement, and then follow as it returns to a more central position. We do not take action, but simply follow what is happening without encouraging or impeding the movement. For the person being followed, the experience is like being accompanied on a journey by someone who is trusted, reliable, and neutral. Movement in the direction of ease is

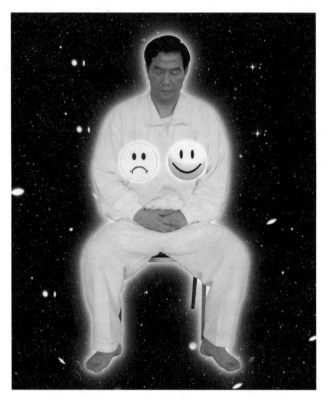

Fig. 5.2. Following the Flow

usually relaxing and comforting, while movement in the direction of discomfort provides valuable information about how tension is being held and about which areas would benefit from more Flow (fig. 5.2).

Unwinding the Knots

Movement can also turn into *unwinding*. Unwinding can take several forms. One type of unwinding occurs when we notice that our awareness is being called in a particular direction, and we explore it. We allow our sense of curiosity to guide us on a completely spontaneous journey. Our mind drops away. Rather than moving consciously, we feel as if we are being moved by something larger than ourselves. It is an adventure that may take us to places we have never been before. These spontaneous movements may take the form of twitches or wave-like motions through the body. When this happens, simply allow the energy to flow until it is complete. This kind of unwinding can be freeing, refreshing, and sometimes even euphoric. We might also feel a little tired at the end, just as we do after some of our more active holidays.

Another type of unwinding occurs when we move with a structure until it reaches the limit of its range. We take care not to force the structure to cross that limit, simply holding it at the boundary and waiting patiently until a shift occurs (fig. 5.3). Typically, the area of tension softens and the boundary dissolves, increasing both our range of motion and our sense of fluidity. As it does so, emotions often release and thought patterns shift. Unwinding is more "active" than the following described above. In unwinding we follow the movement to its limit and then actively invite it to stay at that position (without returning or continuing on its repetitive loop) until a change occurs and a new form of movement unfolds.

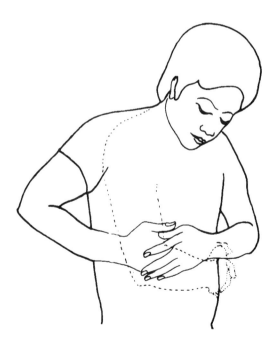

Fig. 5.3. Unwinding the knots

Noticing the Signs of Release during Unwinding

As tension in an area begins to unwind, it is common to notice the following signs of release.

- Softening/spreading/lengthening
- Smoother movement, greater range, more symmetry
- Increased fluidity and energy flow
- Emotional release: crying, laughing, shouting (anger/irritation), groaning/yawning, singing
- Temperature changes, vibration, or pulsation
- Dissolving of thought patterns and stories; allowing new perceptions or ideas

Since the fascia throughout the body is connected, as one area releases, shifts in other more distant parts of the body may occur.

APPLYING CONCEPTS OF FLOW TO THE TAI CHI CHI KUNG PRACTICE

Tai Chi practitioners will already be familiar with the habits of listening, following, and unwinding discussed above. In Tai Chi, we are always listening . . . listening with our feet, with our hands, and with our energy senses. When we play Push Hands with our fellow practitioners, we also listen with our hearts so that no one is injured, and so that we can help our partners improve their skills. We also learn how to follow in Tai Chi, matching a partner perfectly—moving as she moves without amplifying or hindering her movement. We are skillful at knowing when a partner has reached the limit of her range, and understand that it is at that place that change often occurs: the point of greatest vulnerability is often the place of greatest opportunity. Unwinding happens when we are no longer aware of who is leading and who is following.

In this state of interplay, we release our mental body, let go of any thoughts, and sink into the shifting energy. Movement seems to emerge from the joint field rather than from one person or the other. If we are willing to relax completely at this point, we find ourselves moving and responding in ways that we might not have expected or predicted. Emotions may arise—such as fear, frustration, or exhilaration—but they are transient, and we are able to return easily to a calm and centered place. We may receive insights into our patterns and into what we need to do to shift them. As we train in this way, we expand our range on all levels and in all areas of our life.

Push Hands Exercises

To get a sense of how listening, following, and unwinding work, try some simple partner exercises. Because we often sense things more easily in others than we do in ourselves, these exercises effectively prepare us for our work with ourselves. Although Push Hands training is sometimes used for the purpose of developing martial skills, its purpose here is to work with each other to learn the skills that will help us discover more Flow in ourselves and others. Cooperative rather than competitive, we will be working together to learn to listen, follow, and unwind.

Push Hands: Listening

1. Stand facing your partner.
2. Each person takes a step backward with the right foot, so that the left foot is leading. The feet are about shoulder-width apart. Both knees are bent slightly to protect the joints.
3. Place the back of your left hand against the back of your partner's left hand. There should be just enough pressure to make and maintain contact (see fig. 5.4 on page 106).
4. Relax. Listen for the Flow and let the internal movement lead to external motion.
5. When the hands begin to move, continue to listen, keeping the back of your hand in contact with your partner's hand throughout the exercise.

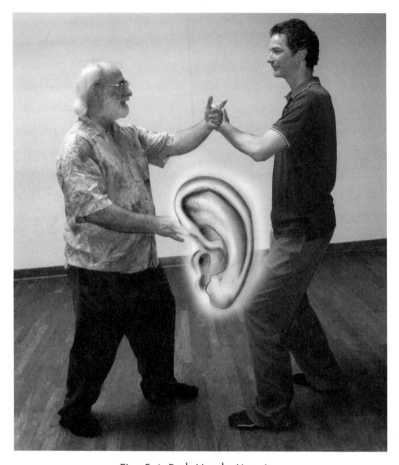

Fig. 5.4. Push Hands: Listening

6. As the hands move, allow your whole body to move with them.

7. What do you notice about your partner? How relaxed and comfortable does he seem? Do you sense that he is tired or vibrant? Does he feel angry, sad, content, or happy?

8. Tune in to your heart and try listening with it. Observe without judgment, just noticing what you notice. When we listen in this way we can receive quite a lot of information.

9. What do you notice about yourself? How is your body? How are your emotions? How are your thoughts? Listen with your heart to yourself. Try to observe without being critical of yourself.

Push Hands: Following

In this exercise, one person leads and the other follows. Decide who will start as leader.

1. With the back of the left hands still touching, both participants should reach out with the right hand to grasp the partner's left elbow. This increase in contact allows us to sense more movement (fig. 5.5).

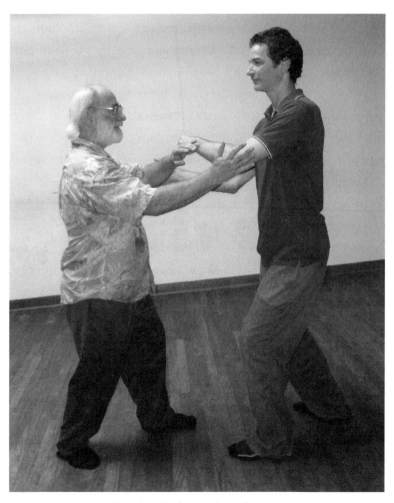

Fig. 5.5. Push Hands: Following

2. The leader begins to allow the Flow to move his left hand. The job of the follower is simply to match the movement without anticipating or slowing it.

3. Switch roles with your partner. Notice the feeling when your partner is in perfect synchrony with you: it may seem as if you are both moving together rather than as if one is leading and the other is following.

Push Hands: Noticing the Direction of Movement

1. Switch roles again. Take the same stance with the left foot leading and the right foot behind. This time, place the palms of both of your hands in contact with your partner's palms (fig. 5.6).

2. When you are the leader, begin by listening. As you move, listen for the quality of your partner's movements. In which directions does she move easily? In which directions does she seem to have difficulty or resistance? Notice that one hand may be moving quite differently than the other.

3. How far can your partner move in the direction of ease? How far can she move in the direction of discomfort? Notice your partner's range of movement in each of those directions. What happens to the quality of movement as she reaches the edge of her limit?

4. When it is your partner's turn to lead and listen, observe your own experience. Notice which movements are easier than others. Feel the difference in the quality of your movement. In some directions, movement may be smooth and fluid; in others, it might feel more jerky or constricted. Notice any thoughts or emotions that arise as your partner explores your limits. What happens as you approach your limit and then as you reach it? You may feel that you tense up or that fear or anger arises. Your partner might not yet be able to tell exactly where your limits are. What happens if you go past your limit? How do you feel? How do you feel toward your partner? How do you feel about yourself?

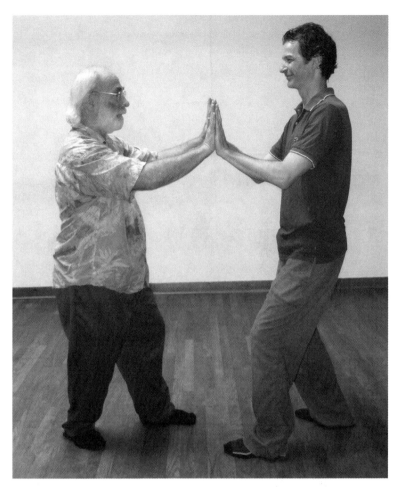

Fig. 5.6. Push Hands: Noticing Direction of Movement

Push Hands: Unwinding

1. As in the exercise above, have the palms of both hands in contact with those of your partner. In this exercise, neither of you is leading.
2. Start with listening from the heart. Relax. Breathe. Let your eyes soften.
3. Allow the movement to begin on its own. Let it unfold. Breathe. Relax.

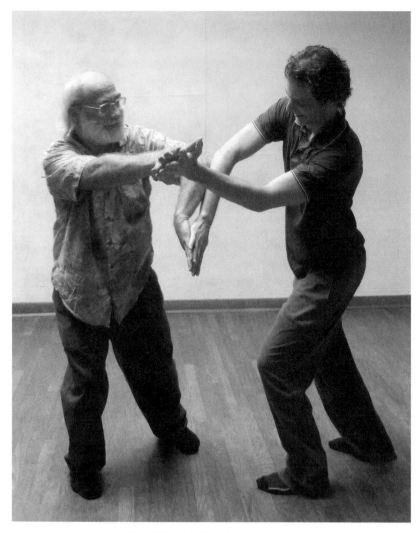

Fig. 5.7. Push Hands: Unwinding

4. You may notice that some patterns repeat again and again and then suddenly move in a new angle or direction (fig. 5.7). There is sometimes a tendency for movement to accelerate. If that happens, invite it to slow. Sometimes movement will stop for a while and then resume on its own. Movement has its own intelligence; the rest periods are a natural part of our integration process. When the movement feels complete, bring the exercise to a close.

BALANCING EMOTIONAL FLOW

Now that you have experienced listening, following, and unwinding with a partner, you can apply these techniques to balancing your own emotional flow. Craniosacral work often addresses emotional flow by focusing on those parts of the body that typically store a lot of emotional energy—the psoas muscle and the belly.

Psoas—The Muscle of the Soul

Structurally, the psoas muscle connects the spine to the legs (fig. 5.8). On the spine, it spans from the twelfth thoracic vertebra (T12) to the fifth lumbar vertebra (L5), then descends through the pelvic region to attach to the top of the femur (thigh bone). This important muscle enables us to lift our legs and therefore affects structural balance, pelvic movement, range of motion in the legs, and the way we walk. In addition to stabilizing the spine, the psoas influences our flexibility, strength, joint mobility, and organs.

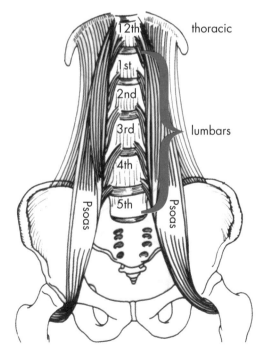

Fig. 5.8. Psoas muscle

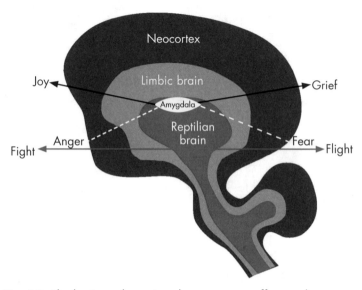

Fig. 5.9. The brain and emotions have a strong effect on the psoas.

Because the psoas is directly connected to the spinal cord and to the reptilian part of the brain through the fascia, it is often the first muscle to contract and the last to release when we experience anger or fear and our system moves into instinctive fight-or-flight reactions. When we are surprised, it is the rapid contraction of the psoas that causes us to "start." The psoas is also activated when we reflexively curl up into a fetal position in times of stress (fig. 5.9).

In ancient days, stress was relatively short term; we either escaped the saber-toothed tiger or we did not. Today, our hectic, high-pressure lifestyle chronically triggers and shortens the psoas but doesn't typically prompt it to lengthen back out, which can lead to back, hip, knee, and sciatic pain (fig. 5.10). In addition to structural issues, a tight psoas impinges on nerves, reduces fluid movement, and hinders full diaphragmatic breathing. Moreover, when the psoas is overactivated, it continually signals the nervous system to be alert for danger. This continuous state of alert exhausts our adrenals and taxes our immune system. Psoas tension is also implicated in digestive issues, menstrual pain, and infertility.

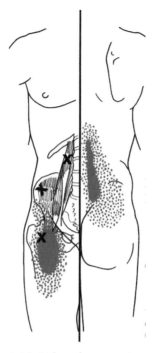

Fig. 5.10. When the psoas is tense,
it causes pain in other places.

Because the psoas is so closely connected to our instinctual survival reactions, and because of its deep location in the body, many people store unresolved emotions or unhealed traumas in this muscle. When we feel criticized (by others or by ourselves), it is often the psoas that reacts by contracting and becoming rigid. Taoists refer to the psoas as the muscle of the soul because of its connection to our deepest essence and core identity.

Relaxing the Psoas Muscle

As we've discovered, the psoas is particularly reactive to fear, anxiety, and anger. When we experience those emotions, the psoas contracts. Because the upper attachments of the psoas are in the same region as the diaphragm, contraction in the psoas affects the diaphragm and causes shallow breathing. By consciously deepening and lengthening our breathing, we relax tension in our diaphragm and release the psoas. As the psoas relaxes and tension dissolves, our emotional blockages begin to melt and dissolve as well.

Other benefits of releasing the psoas include improved circulation of oxygen, blood, and lymph, and improved detoxification as the stress hormones stored in the tissues dissipate. As restrictions dissolve and circulation increases, our tissues are also able to repair themselves more quickly. As Flow increases, we can experience an expanded range of physical motion and greater emotional mobility as well.

Since this muscle wraps the lower tan tien, it also affects our energy flow. The psoas is the only muscle to connect the spine with the legs, so when the psoas is relaxed, it is easier for energy to flow from the earth up the legs and to the spine. And as the downward force of gravity meets the earth and rebounds with each step we take, a resilient psoas can transfer the energy upward, energizing and awakening the spine.

Refreshing Lotus Meditation

Imagine the heart as a red lotus flower and the pericardium (the heat-regulating membrane that encloses the heart) as the lotus pads. Visualize the kidneys as bulbs, similar to the clusters or plexuses where the stems of the pads and the lotus flower join together. In a pond or pool there are usually several lotus plants that join together in a cluster, anchoring in the mud. From the kidneys (kidney bulbs/clusters), visualize roots extending down through the legs into the watery mud of the earth basin.

Through this dreamscape imagery of the body and the lotus merging in nature, sense these qualities of energy in your body. Feel the warm red energy of the heart connecting with the red and yellow/gold from the sun above. Likewise, sense the cool, blue water energy of the kidneys merging with the refreshing blue water energy from the earth.

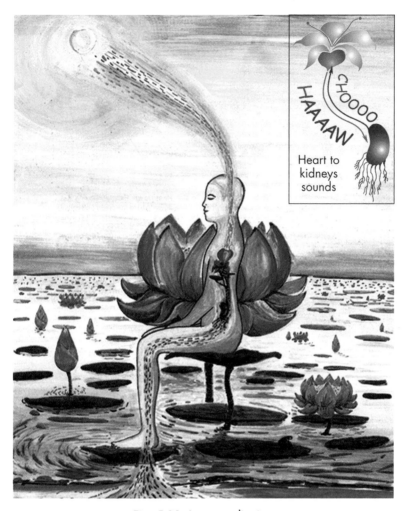

Fig. 5.11. Lotus meditation

 Yin Breathing

Strong emotional reactions are associated with erratic or strained breathing patterns. Natural breathing smoothes out emotional swings by quieting the mind and retraining our nervous system to relax. Yin breathing accentuates this process even further, bringing us to meditative states of tranquility.

Yin breathing assists us in releasing psoas tension and the emotions held there. In addition, the meditative state induced by yin breathing also helps to rebalance our emotions.

1. Find a comfortable position either sitting or lying.
2. Align your body so that your head is in line with your heart and hips.
3. Take a snapshot of how you feel physically, emotionally, and mentally.
4. Begin natural breathing, inhaling and exhaling through your nose. Breathe into the solar plexus area to relax the psoas.
5. Notice your inhalations and exhalations. Invite your breath to deepen and slow, becoming smoother and more even.
6. Slowly begin to lengthen your exhalation until it is twice the length of your inhalation.
7. Continue slowing your breath until your inhalation is around 7 seconds and your exhalation lasts about 14 seconds.
8. Do 9 rounds and then allow your breathing to return to normal.
9. Notice how you feel and what has changed.

Listening with the Heart to Your Psoas Muscle

Since the psoas often holds emotional trauma in the form of tension, physical work with this muscle can be intense. Yang-style deep tissue work can often be effective in working with the psoas but in some cases may create more constriction as a defensive reaction. In the following exercise, we will take the yin approach of inviting rather than insisting that the psoas open and release.

For this exercise, lie comfortably with a pillow underneath your knees to relax the lower back and abdomen.

1. Find the psoas release points approximately two inches to the side and one inch below the belly button on each side. Palpate gently in the area on both sides until you sense some tension or a magnetic whorl of energy that pulls you into it.

2. Choose one side to work with first and let go of the other side.

3. Take a moment to smile to your psoas, sending it love, comfort, and safety. Invite it to relax and open.

4. Use the index and middle fingers of one hand to slowly and gently make contact with the point you palpated in step 1. The job of this hand is to remain relaxed and to listen.

5. Place your second hand on top of the first. The job of the second hand is to apply any pressure if needed (fig. 5.12).

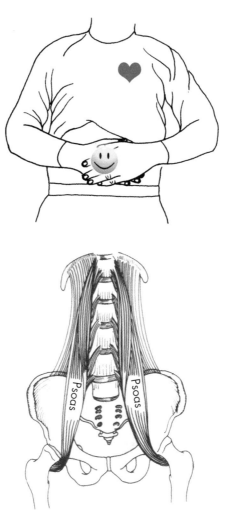

Fig. 5.12. Smiling to the psoas

6. Placing your awareness into the fingers of the first hand, allow them to listen to the psoas. Do nothing except listen. Listen with your heart for the story and message of the psoas. Listen with patience, with compassion, and with presence.

7. What story does your psoas need to tell? What does your psoas need to feel safe? To relax? To release?

8. Wait until the psoas has finished its story. You will know it is done when it softens. Then repeat on the second side.

As you continue to rest and integrate the story of the psoas, notice what feels different in your legs, pelvis, and spine as you lie down. Continue to sense the changes as you sit and stand up. Because we use the psoas to walk, also notice if anything has changed in your gait.

Caution: Because of the strong relationship among our physical, mental, and emotional bodies, it is important not to force or rush changes. Working too deeply, forcefully, or quickly to release physical tension may cause trauma or cause previous traumas to surface. In Craniosacral Work, we say that if we go slowly, we give the body and energy field time to respond rather than react. By allowing time for our systems to get used to what is happening—time to relax and soften—we can often go deeper than would be otherwise possible.

Psoas Muscle Release

This exercise provides another opportunity to release the psoas and increase the flow of emotions that may have accumulated there.

For this exercise, it may be helpful to have a chair nearby, or to work near a wall for added stability.

1. Start by sitting cross-legged to warm up your hip joints.
2. Keeping your back straight, make small circles in a clockwise direction with your torso (fig. 5.13).

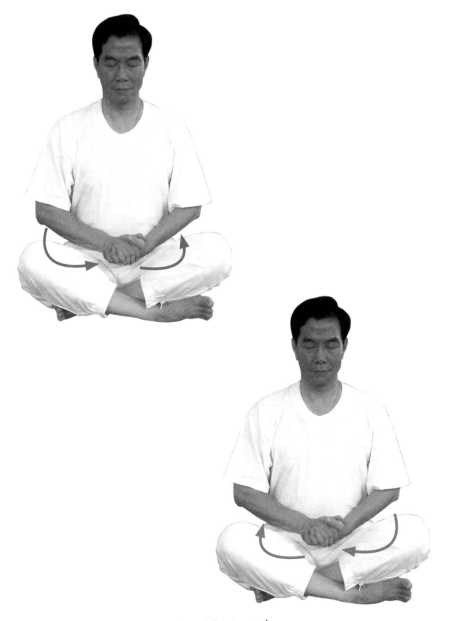

Fig. 5.13. Hip circles

3. Rotate 18 times, slowly increasing the size of the circle.
4. Reverse direction and rotate 18 times in a counterclockwise direction. Start with small circles and gradually increase their size.

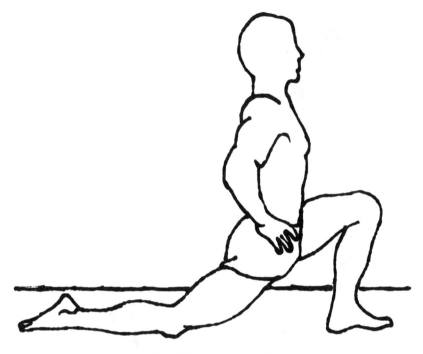

Fig. 5.14. Psoas stretch

5. Now, come to a runner's lunge with the front knee directly over the ankle and the back knee resting on the floor (fig. 5.14). (If you are on a hard floor, place a towel or yoga mat underneath to provide some cushioning for your knee.)

6. The focus is on stretching and opening the psoas in your back leg. To do so, your back knee should be behind your hips. Keep your spine upright with your head aligned directly over your hips.

7. Once you have found the position, breathe. Smile into your psoas and invite it to relax.

8. As you settle into this position, you will notice layers of tension in the various muscles peeling away like layers of an onion.

9. Notice any tension you are holding in your pelvis and invite it to relax as well.

10. Listen to your psoas. Notice what thoughts or emotions or physical sensations come up as you hold this position.

11. Use the chair or the wall to stabilize yourself, if necessary, so you can sink deeper.

12. Allow your awareness to drop deep into the psoas muscle. Follow the tension to its deep core and smile into whatever is blocking Flow. Sense it softening. As it does so, the muscle may start unwinding and shaking. Rather than tensing up to stop that shaking, soften. Relax into the movement and let the waves of energy move through your body, releasing both local and general restrictions.

13. If possible, stay in this position for 5 minutes, allowing yourself to shake and realign as necessary. Keep coming back to your breath, the invitation to relax, and the Inner Smile you are beaming to the psoas. If necessary, take breaks and return to the position.

14. Once you are done, repeat on the other side.

Note on application to Tai Chi: In addition to releasing our emotions, this psoas stretch is an excellent exercise for helping us to improve our Tai Chi foundations. Because our hips and psoas muscles are tight, many of us find it difficult to get fully into even the basic Tai Chi postures. As you settle into this position, notice the alignment of your torso. Rather than leaning forward, make sure that your head is in alignment with your heart and hips. This change will allow the psoas to lengthen even more in the back leg. Invite your hips to face directly forward and let your tailbone sink toward the earth.

Because of lower back and hip issues, many people do not sink the kua of their front leg and therefore cannot put 70 percent of the weight on the front leg without leaning forward and throwing off their alignment. As you relax into the postures, gradually release and drop the hip of the front leg so that it is level with the other hip. This deepens the kua and stabilizes the pelvis. If you press down on the foot of your front leg, you can then feel earth energy travel up the leg, through the pelvis to the other leg, then down to the knee of the back leg and into the earth. Thus, this position is useful for feeling the energy flow through the lower limbs as well as learning to close the kua of the front leg and open the kua of the back leg. Over time, you will notice that this exercise changes and benefits your entire Tai Chi practice.

Releasing Stored Emotions from the Belly

Like the psoas, the belly is a place that stores many kinds of energy; it is, in fact, a doorway between our physical, emotional, mental, and energy bodies. All the energy channels that create and sustain the physical body emerge from and return to the belly. We know that we hold emotions in our belly as well: when we are nervous, we get butterflies in the stomach; when we are stressed we get stomachaches; and when we are shocked we may feel as if we were punched in the gut. When we release tension from the belly, our emotions and our chi are able to flow more freely. Then the ocean of chi can heal and restore the body to its original wholeness and health.

We can free the abdomen from tension and stored emotions with breathing exercises, Chi Nei Tsang self-massage, and Chi Kung. Sometimes we may link the emotional and physical releases to memories of specific past events. Other times, we may not have a clear understanding why certain emotions surface as tension subsides in our body. Either way, allow what rises to the surface to be released and invite peace and harmony to flow in and fill the space that is created.

 ## Empty Force Breathing

To help prepare us for our work with the abdomen, it is very helpful to do a few rounds of Empty Force Breathing to increase circulation in the tissues and release adhesions in the organs.

1. Stand with your feet shoulder-width apart and your knees and shoulders relaxed.
2. Take a deep breath in through the nose.

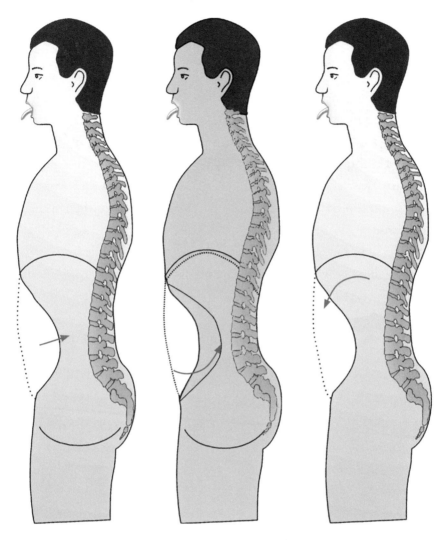

Fig. 5.15. Empty Force Breathing

3. Exhale completely through the mouth with your tongue out.
4. After a full exhalation, contract your abdomen, drawing it up toward the diaphragm, then rolling it out and down (fig. 5.15). Roll your belly 9 times, creating a vacuum in the abdomen.
5. After the ninth roll, release your belly and take a long slow deep inhalation through your nose and repeat steps 3–5.
6. Do 3 complete rounds of 9 rolls each.

Unwinding the Flow Using Chi Nei Tsang Self-Massage

Chi Nei Tsang means working with the energy (*chi*) of the internal (*nei*) organs (*tsang*). By working with the organs, Chi Nei Tsang can clear physical toxins, release emotional holding stored in the organs, and unwind mental blockages. In ancient times, monks used this practice to detoxify, strengthen, and refine their bodies so that they would be able to sustain the high vibrational energy necessary for their spiritual practices.

This Chi Nei Tsang exercise can be done seated while leaning forward slightly, or lying face up with a pillow under your knees to reduce tension in the abdomen.

1. Spend a moment to take a baseline snapshot of how you are physically, emotionally, and mentally.
2. Use the index and middle fingers of one hand to gently trace your navel, sensing the skin and underlying structures.
3. Next, slightly widen the diameter of the circle around the navel and repeat, sensing for areas of fluidity and areas of tension.
4. After you have completed the second circuit, return to an area of tension.
5. Touch your belly with the index and middle fingers of one hand, and relax any tension in the fingers. This is your sensing or yin hand.
6. Rest your second hand on top of the first (fig. 5.16). This is the active or yang hand; it can be used to apply slight pressure as needed. Using the yang hand to apply pressure allows the yin hand to remain receptive and able to perceive more.
7. Listen with your fingers and your heart for the movement of the tissues. Explore.
8. Notice the direction of ease and the direction of discomfort.
9. When you become aware of the direction of ease, follow the tissues

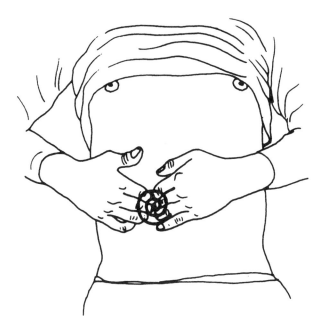

Fig. 5.16. Chi Nei Tsang self-massage

in that direction until they reach their limit. Rest for a moment, then follow the tissues back toward the starting position. Repeat 2 or more times.

10. The next time, when the tissues reach their limit and begin their return, hold them at the boundary with kindness and compassion.

11. Sense the dynamic unwinding movement of the tissues as they adjust. Continue to hold them at the boundary. Within a few seconds, the tissues will go neutral and become still as they reorganize. A few seconds later, follow them as they begin to move again. Notice that the pattern of movement will often be different after they have "rebooted." You may also notice that the range of movement is larger than previously and that you feel a sense of expansion and relaxation.

Once a release occurs in the direction of ease, there is usually a change in the direction of discomfort as well. It is possible to do this type of release work by moving directly into the direction of discomfort, but it is often more challenging, and there can be more resistance to letting go.

12. Relax and shake out your hands and take three deep breaths. During this gentle process, you may have observed emotions and thoughts coming to the surface in addition to physical sensations. What has changed physically and mentally for you since the snapshot you took at the beginning of this exercise?

Note: As in Chi Kung, minimum effort often produces maximum effect in Chi Nei Tsang: more pressure is not necessarily better or more helpful. The lighter the pressure, the less tension there will be in your hands. The more relaxed your hands, the more they can sense. Additionally, the lighter the pressure, the lower the likelihood that you will cause your system to become reactive, defensive, or resistant.

People often feel lighter and freer after the Chi Nei Tsang self-massage. They feel more fluid, flexible, and alive. This is because the fascial layers of the abdomen store and conduct chi. When our chi is low, the fascia become dry and hard. This restricts our movement, and we feel stiff and inflexible. By opening up the fascia and releasing the flow of chi, we restore health, ground our emotions, and stabilize our mental body.

BALANCING THE MENTAL FLOWS
Leveraging the Mental and Emotional Connection

As we discussed earlier, the interconnectivity of our physical, emotional, and mental bodies offers us many options for our inner work. Sometimes an indirect approach can be extremely effective. In the last section, we used physical exercises to open and release our emotions in order to encourage our emotional flow. In this section, we will use exercises typically focused on balancing our emotions to harmonize our mental body and facilitate mental flow.

The idea that emotions "just happen" to us has been a commonly accepted belief for several centuries in the Western world. More recently, the link between emotions and our thoughts has become better understood. Cognitive behavior therapy, for example, emphasizes the important role of thoughts in influencing our emotions. Our thoughts and perspectives about situations affect the emotions that we experience in those situations.

Yet the relationship between thought and emotion is a two-way interaction: while our thoughts can influence our emotions, our emotions likewise affect our thoughts—our decision-making abilities as well as our cognition. If you reflect on your own life experience, it will probably not take long for you to recall instances in which strong emotions affected your perceptions and ability to think clearly.

The initial reaction to a situation often comes from emotions and feelings. This initial emotional reaction actually influences the analytical thoughts that follow. Evolutionarily, our immediate emotional reactions helped us to survive when the need for quick reflexes did not leave space or time to think through a complete assessment of the situation. Although rational analytical thinking is valued in today's society, our systems are still wired to use our emotions to evaluate situations and to guide our behavior in many circumstances. This dynamic suggests that cultivating emotional balance will have a positive effect on your mental body and on your ability to optimize outcomes.

Engaging our Back-to-the-Body Wisdom

In our thought-focused culture, we often we spend relatively too much time in our heads; the simple breathing and stretching postures of Chi Kung and meditation are useful in bringing us back into the body. As the exercises harmonize our physical and emotional aspects, the mind clears and settles as well.

This is an easy and valuable way to shift our negative thoughts, which can be just as damaging as our negative emotions. Once we become aware of those negative thought patterns, it can still be a challenge to change old habits. Anyone who has ever tried not thinking about something knows how difficult that can be. A different, and sometimes easier approach, is to transform the negative emotions and then invite in the positive mental and emotional qualities.

The benefits of doing so are significant. When we are thinking or worrying too much, our brain can consume as much 80 percent of our energy. This does not leave very much energy for anything else. If you can use your Chi Kung practices to balance your emotions and quiet your mind, then you will have more energy available for growth and spiritual development.

To help balance your emotions, try the following Laughter Chi Kung exercise.

Laughter Chi Kung

Laughter is a natural way to release stress as well as circulate more oxygen and blood through the body. Laughter Chi Kung helps direct those benefits to release physical tension, move the emotions, and clear the mind.

Sounds are powerful in transforming energy. The sound "Ha" generates and improves the flow of chi, promoting a sense of clarity, well-being and happiness. The vibration that is created during laughter activates the gut brain in the lower tan tien and the whole abdominal area. This in turn helps to clear and release all the organs. As the laughter vibration stimulates the diaphragm, our breath deepens, increasing circulation and reducing stress on the heart. As the vibration moves through the heart and thymus, it boosts our immune systems.

1. Take another snapshot of how you feel physically, emotionally, and mentally in this moment.
2. Take a moment to think of something funny or amusing, then invite your mind to drop down to your lower abdomen.
3. Take a full deep breath in through your nose.
4. Lean forward slightly and exhale completely while making the sound "HaHaHa" (fig. 5.17).

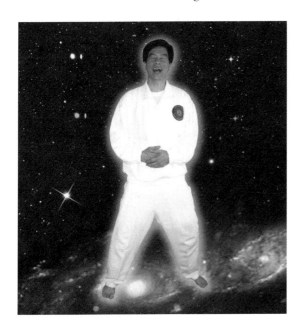

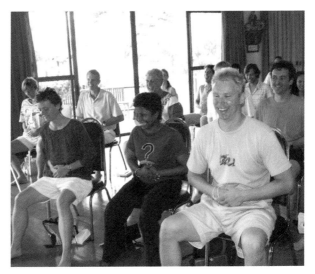

Fig. 5.17. Laughter Chi Kung

The more genuine the laughter, the more effective it is at clearing and balancing. However, if you are doing this exercise at a time when real laughter is not accessible to you, then it is still beneficial to "fake it until you make it."

5. Repeat this exercise 3–5 times. Feel the vibration in the tan tien and heart each time.

6. After the last repetition, pause after the full exhalation.

7. Inhale slowly and smoothly through your nose and resume regular breathing.

8. Gather and store the chi in your lower tan tien.

9. Take another snapshot of your well-being and notice what has shifted for you.

The Six Healing Sounds for Mental Balance

Negative emotions are stored in the body's organs. Over time, the accumulation of negativity erodes organ health and also affects our thinking. The Six Healing Sounds meditation is an alchemical process that transforms the negative energy stuck in the organs. Once that energy is flowing freely, it also transmutes our thinking. Although the focus in Six Healing Sounds is often on the emotions, this time we will explore how the practice shifts the state of our mental body.

Note: When doing these practices, it is common to yawn, burp, or pass wind. These actions are a sign that energy is moving through the system and are considered to be beneficial.

The Lungs' Sound—Metal Element

The lungs' sound transforms sadness into courage.

1. Sit on the edge of your chair with your back straight and your feet shoulder-width apart.

2. Rest your hands on your lungs with your eyes closed. Smile to your lungs until you make a good connection with them.

3. Imagine that you are looking into the lobes of your lungs, moving your eyes right and left 21 times. Look for any grief or sadness there and invite them to release. The third or sixth time you do this step,

look into the left and right hemispheres of your brain. Delete any negative programming related to grief or sadness.

4. On your next inhalation, open your eyes and raise both hands over your head with the palms facing up and fingers pointing toward each other. Look up (fig. 5.18).

5. Close your jaws so that the teeth touch gently and make the sound "sss-s-s-s-s-s" as you exhale slowly.

6. Feel the metal vibration clearing your lungs of toxins and your emotional body of grief.

7. Inhale as you scoop up white light and pour it down through your crown to your lungs as you exhale, lowering your arms until they face your chest.

8. Smile and radiate a pure white light to fill your lungs, transforming

Lungs: clarity

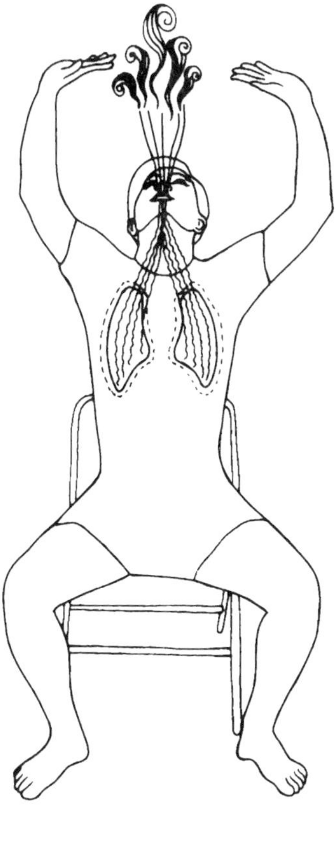

Fig. 5.18.
The Lungs' Sound

any remaining sadness or grief into courage. Continue to feel the sound vibrating into your lungs.

9. See your lungs glowing with the clear white light of the metal element. Invite the quality of clarity into your mental body.

10. Practice the lungs' metal element exercise (steps 3–10) a total of 3 or 6 times.

The Kidneys' Sound—Water Element

The kidneys' sound transforms fear into gentleness and calmness.

1. Sit comfortably, resting your hands on your kidneys with your eyes closed.

2. Smile down to your kidneys until you feel you are in touch with them.

3. Imagine that you are looking into your kidneys, moving your eyes right and left 21 times. Look for any fear there and invite it to release. The third or sixth time you do this step, look into the left and right hemispheres of your brain. Delete any negative programming related to fear.

4. Bring your legs close together so that the ankles and knees touch. Clasp your hands around your knees and straighten your arms by leaning backward slightly (fig. 5.19). On your next inhalation, draw your knees in and up slightly until your heels are off the floor; only the Bubbling Spring point at the base of your toes should be touching the ground. Lean slightly forward with a rounded back and look straight ahead.

5. Round your lips and exhale the sound "choo-oo-oo-oo."

6. Feel the water vibration cleansing your kidneys of debris and your emotional body of fear.

7. On your next inhale, separate your legs and scoop blue light up and pour it over your crown to your kidneys on the exhale.

8. Place your palms on your kidneys and radiate blue light to them,

Kidneys: wisdom and insight

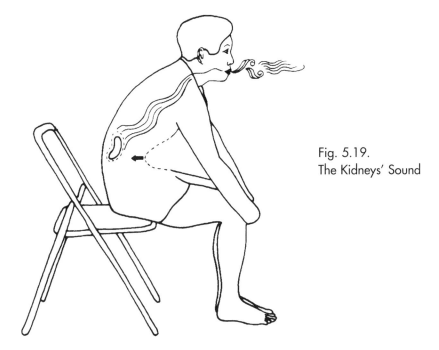

Fig. 5.19.
The Kidneys' Sound

transforming any remaining fear into gentleness and calmness. Continue to feel the sound vibrating your kidneys.

9. Smile and see your kidneys glowing with the deep blue light of the water element. Let your mind open to wisdom and new insights.

10. Practice the water exercise 3 or 6 times.

The Liver's Sound—Wood Element

The liver's sound transforms anger into kindness.

1. Sit with your back straight and your hands resting on your liver— under the right side of your ribcage.

2. Smile to your liver until you can connect with it.

3. Imagine that you are looking into your liver, moving your eyes right and left 21 times. Look for any anger or irritation there and invite them to release. The third or sixth time you do this step, look into

the left and right hemispheres of your brain. Delete any negative programming related to anger or jealousy.

4. On your next inhalation, extend your hands out to your sides with your palms up. Continue to raise your hands upward until you can clasp them over your head and interlace your fingers (fig. 5.20).
5. Lean slightly to the left and look up.
6. Exhale the sound "sh-h-h-h-h-h-h."
7. Feel the wood vibration detoxifying your liver and your emotional body of anger, irritation, frustration, or jealousy.
8. After you have completely exhaled, separate your hands. As you inhale, scoop green light up and pour it down to your liver on the exhale.
9. Place your hands on your liver and radiate green light to fill it, transforming any remaining anger into kindness. Continue to feel the sound vibrating your liver.

Liver: good decision making

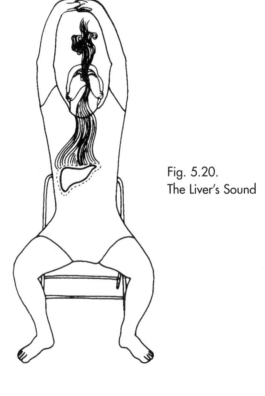

Fig. 5.20.
The Liver's Sound

10. Smile and see your liver glowing with the deep green light of the wood element. Sense how easily you can make good decisions and carry them out.
11. Practice the wood element exercise 3 or 6 times.

The Heart's Sound—Fire Element

The heart's sound transforms impatience and cruelty into joy.

1. Place your hands on your heart while you sit on the edge of your chair with your back straight.
2. Smile into your heart until you can sense it.
3. Imagine that you are looking into your heart, moving your eyes right and left 21 times. Look for any hatred, cruelty, or impatience there and invite them to release. The third or sixth time you do this step, look into the left and right hemispheres of your brain. Delete any negative programming related to hatred, cruelty, or impatience.
4. On your next inhalation, extend your hands out to your sides with your palms up and let them rise until you can clasp them over your head and interlace your fingers (see fig. 5.21 on page 136).
5. Lean slightly to the right and look up.
6. Exhale the sound "haw-w-w-w-w-w" with a wide open mouth.
7. Feel the fire vibration cleansing your heart and your emotional body of impatience, hatred, and cruelty.
8. Once you have exhaled fully, separate your hands. On your next inhale, scoop red light up and pour it from your crown to your heart on your exhale.
9. Hold your hands in front of your heart and radiate red light to fill it with love, joy, and happiness. Feel the heart continue to vibrate with the sound.
10. Smile and see your heart glowing with the rich red light of the fire

Heart: creativity

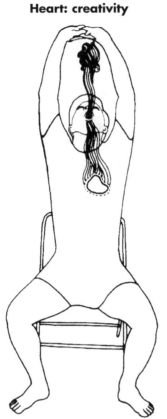

Fig. 5.21.
The Heart's Sound

element. Feel the creative aspect of your mind awaken and begin to express itself.

11. Practice the fire element exercise 3 or 6 times.

The Spleen's Sound—Earth Element

The spleen's sound transforms anxiety into fairness, openness, and trust.

1. Sit with your back straight, resting your hands on your spleen—to the left of the sternum, underneath the rib cage (fig. 5.22).
2. Smile to your spleen until you feel it respond.
3. Imagine that you are looking into your spleen, moving your eyes right

Spleen: intellect and focus

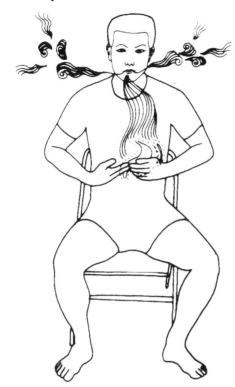

Fig. 5.22.
The Spleen's Sound

and left 21 times. Look for any worry, anxiety, or mistrust there and invite these emotions to release. The third or sixth time you do this step, look into the left and right hemispheres of your brain. Delete any negative programming related to worry, anxiety, or mistrust.

4. Place the three middle fingers of each hand on the spleen. Inhale. Press gently and make the sound "who-o-o-o-o-o" as you exhale. This sound should come from the chest rather than the mouth.

5. Feel the earth sound vibrating the spleen, stomach, and pancreas.

6. On your next inhale, scoop yellow light up and pour it through your spleen and stomach on the exhale.

7. Bring your hands to your spleen and/or stomach.

8. Smile and radiate yellow light, along with the qualities of fairness, openness, and trust, to the spleen and stomach. Feel the spleen's sound continue to vibrate the organs.

9. See your spleen glowing with the nurturing yellow light of the earth element. Feel your intellect and ability to focus become sharper.

10. Practice the earth element exercise a total of 3 or 6 times.

The Triple Warmer's Sound

The Triple Warmer regulates the temperatures of the three tan tiens and also balances the energies activated by all of the six healing sounds. It helps the entire system to relax more deeply.

1. Lie down or lean backward into your chair with your feet stretched out in front of you (fig. 5.23).

2. Smile into your three centers.

3. As you inhale, gather chi and raise your hands over your head. As you exhale, slowly bring your hands down in front of your body,

Triple Warmer: connection

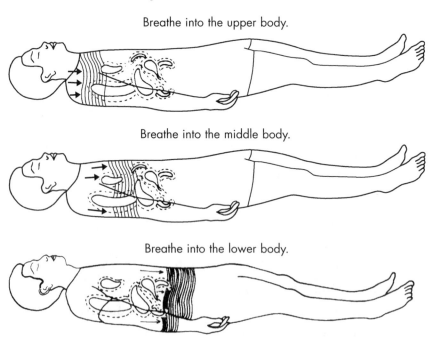

Fig. 5.23. The Triple Warmer's sound

moving the energy from your crown to your feet as you make the sound "hee-e-e-e-e-e."

4. Feel the sound vibrating your three tan tiens as any excess heat flows toward the earth.

5. In the space that is created, rest and absorb cosmic energy. Feel your mind quiet and relaxed, connected with your body, emotions, and mind.

6. Practice the Triple Warmer exercise 3 or 6 times.

ACCESSING GREATER HARMONY

Through the Chi Kung and Craniosacral Work practices in this chapter, we have been learning how to notice and be present with what *is*. We have improved our awareness of the waves of emotion and thought that arise, and are better able to choose which waves can move through us and subside, and which ones we want to ride, encourage, and enjoy. With skill and wisdom, we are able to use the power of our

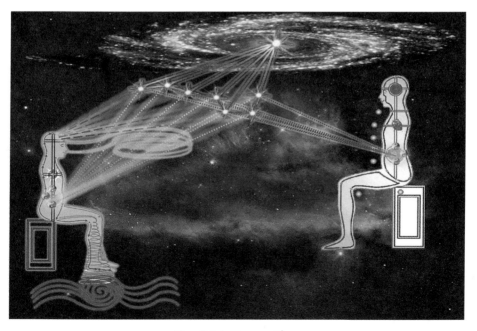

Fig. 5.24. Greater Flow

emotions and intentions rather than become overwhelmed by them.

As we go forward, we will find that increasing Flow in these areas increases our ability to sense the movement of chi itself, because we know how to relax, release, and focus. Furthermore, the harmony that we are able to access and experience through the Chi Kung practices is critical to our spiritual growth. When we make harmonizing our inner world a priority, harmony with the external world comes much easier. The Tao teaches us that our experience of the outer world is a reflection of the world inside us.

PART THREE

Spiritual Flow

In the preceding chapters we increased the Flow of our fluids, bones, and tissues in order to create more fluidity in our physical, emotional, and mental bodies. Especially for newcomers to Chi Kung and energy work, it can be both helpful and reassuring to start with these more familiar aspects of ourselves. Awakening, generating, and sustaining Flow on these levels is not only beneficial in and of itself but is also important in connecting to the energy moving within ourselves, our communities, and the cosmos.

Next we will explore the energetics and spirituality of our internal structures, deepening our understanding of our parts before we open our awareness to the Whole.

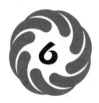

Everything Is Energy

In school, children learn about Albert Einstein's famous equation $E=mc^2$ (Energy = mass x the speed of light squared). This simple, yet profound, equation tells us that everything is energy (fig. 6.1). The equation also describes the recipe for the relationship between energy and matter (or mass).

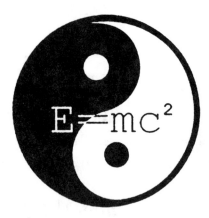

Fig. 6.1. Everything is energy.

Energy can turn into mass (or matter) and mass can turn into energy. Light in motion is what makes that alchemical transformation possible. In Taoism, the physical body is the mass; the fire from our lower tan tien, kidneys, and heart is the light that transforms mass into chi/energy. As we advance in our practices and expand our skills, we can also connect with Dark Matter, which makes up 90 percent of the universe and the cosmic violet light of the sun and stars. These greater sources of mass and light enable us to access even more energy.

WISDOM IN THE BONES

To help us attune to these more subtle forms of mass, light, and movement, we first go back to the basics. The higher we want to go, the more stable and secure our foundations need to be. In Taoism, the foundation is our bones. Bones are the most enduring parts of ourselves, lasting hundreds of thousands of years. Long after we have made our transition, our bones will still be here to tell the stories of our lives. They hold our lineage and enormous wisdom. Many ancient cultures had charnel houses where the bones of the ancestors were preserved and honored (fig. 6.2).

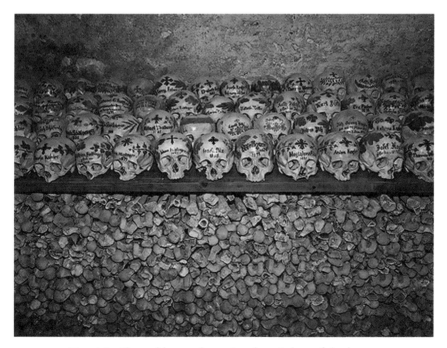

Fig. 6.2. Charnel house: honoring the wisdom of the bones

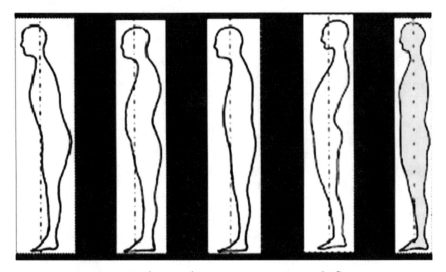

Fig. 6.3. Aligning the structure to optimize chi flow

In Taoist practice, the health and strength of the bones are governed by the kidneys, which are said to be the keepers of our ancestral memory. Biomedical studies in the West show that the anatomical kidneys are directly connected to the brain stem—the ancient reptilian part of the brain, which is the repository of wisdom that is millions of years old.

To access this wisdom, communication pathways must be open. We can tell if the pathways are open by feeling the flow of chi. One of the major impediments to the flow of chi is the misalignment of our physical structure (fig. 6.3). When the skeletal structure is out of alignment due to injury, tension, or poor habits, the chi has more difficulty moving. Craniosacral practitioners keep in mind an ancient Taoist saying that you can't get the head right without the getting the heart right, and you can't get the heart right without getting the sacrum right. Consciously remembering to align the head, heart, and sacrum is enormously helpful for improving energy flow.

Charging the Bones

As we talk about the bones and energy, it is also worth mentioning that our bones are electrically charged. When put under mechanical stress (from pressure for example), electrical polarization occurs, creating what is called a piezoelectric charge. Piezoelectricity regulates bone adaptation and growth. In response to mechanical stress from exercise, our bones actually increase mass and density. In the absence of such stress, our bones shrink and become more fragile. Measurements of bone density in astronauts note small but measurable bone loss in a matter of hours in a gravity-free environment. Chi Kung is valuable for strengthening the bones and for increasing the electrical current that runs through them.

Bones are not only charged with electrical energy but are also highly conductive to vibration. Sound and light waves activate the energy of the bones and increase the chi flowing through them. Chanting, music, ultrasound, infrared, and sunlight are all good ways to amplify the energy that is contained in these deep layers of our being. Then all we need to do is to listen to their wisdom.

Sensing the Energy in Our Bones

Some Chi Kung students become discouraged because they do not think they can feel energy. Everyone has the natural capacity to feel energy, however, and everyone can practice in order to become more skilled at sensing and directing it.

One easy way to sense our energy is to imagine the fuel gauge of a car (fig. 6.4). If we were to ask ourselves how much energy we have in

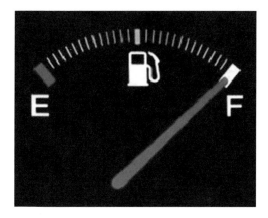

Fig. 6.4. Sensing energy

the moment, would that gauge be on empty, half-way, or full? If you can answer that question, then you can sense your own energy. Chi Kung practices simply refine and deepen your perceptive abilities.

Another good way to sense your energy is to increase it by shaking your bones. Try the following exercise, then feel the chi running through your body.

Shaking the Bones

1. Stand with your feet shoulder-width apart and your knees slightly bent so the energy can move through your joints.
2. Bring your hands in front of you with the elbows bent and touching the sides of your ribs.
3. Let your palms face downward and begin to shake your wrists. Keep your elbows tucked so that the movement in the wrists is accentuated. Shake them about 18 times.
4. Then turn your palms upward and shake your wrists another 18 times. Keep your elbows close to your body and let your wrists be relaxed, flopping back and forth.
5. Let your elbows relax away from your body and turn your palms to face each other.
6. Close your eyes. Can you feel the energy moving through your arms to your fingers? You may feel warmth, tingling, or a sense of movement. You are sensing your chi.
7. You can continue this exercise by allowing your hands to rest comfortably by your sides, leaving some space between your arms and your body to open up the armpit. Bend your knees slightly.
8. Begin to bounce gently on your heels, sending vibration up your legs and spine to your head. Bounce 18 or 36 times, then rest. Close your eyes. Feel the chi running through your entire body.

Bones Affect Our Mood and Memory

Gerard Karsenty, a French geneticist and physician, spent decades exploring the role of osteocalcin, a protein found in high concentrations in bones. He found that osteocalcin regulates important processes throughout the body and facilitates direct communication from the bones to the brain. This finding supported his theory that bones have a larger role in our bodies than just providing an internal framework.

In research with mice, Karsenty showed that osteocalcin in the bones regulated blood sugar and male fertility. He also demonstrated that mice that did not manufacture osteocalcin were anxious and depressed, and also exhibited limited spatial memory. This suggests that bones play a role in both emotions and memory, at least in mice. In pregnant mice, the mother's osteocalcin also impacted fetal development.

Although he has not yet confirmed his hypothesis, Karsenty believes that higher bone mass would be linked to higher osteocalcin production. If this is true, then anything that increases bone density would positively affect mood, memory, and male fertility. If this theory proves correct, it would support the benefits that result from Chi Kung exercises such as Bone Marrow or Iron Shirt Chi Kung.

BONE MOBILITY AND MOTILITY

In addition to aligning, strengthening, and charging our bones, we also need to ensure that they move freely. Movement includes both mobility and motility. In this context, mobility is the ability of the structure to move or be moved. Motility is the inherent, spontaneous movement of the structures without conscious volition. In both cases, the ideal is to have a full and balanced range of motion.

Earlier, we saw that the motility of the sacrum was influenced by the movement of the occiput via the dural tube and spinal cord connection. We discovered that we could consciously mobilize the sacrum through our Chi Kung exercises, which provide an effective way to stimulate the pumping of cerebrospinal fluid—a major conduit for chi in the central nervous system.

The motility of the cranial bones, however, has been somewhat controversial. In the past, Western medicine assumed that the bones in the skull fused after infancy and therefore stopped moving. In part, this idea came from examining the skull after death when the bones had become dehydrated and hard. However, in the early 1900s, Dr. William Garner Sutherland was the first Western doctor to perceive subtle motion in the bones. His research over eighty years demonstrated the inherent motility of the cranial bones: in living, breathing humans, the sutures are flexible and adaptable to allow that motion. Over the years, cranial bone motion in humans and animals has been well-documented by numerous research studies including studies by NASA.[1] All Craniosacral Work rests upon the basic fact of cranial bone motion and endeavors to harmonize the motility of the cranial bones, and thereby optimize the circulation of the cerebrospinal fluid.

In figure 6.5 we see a Beauchene skull, which is a specially prepared disarticulated skull showing the spaciousness in the sutures while preserving the relative position of the bones. This "exploded" skull is used in the study of anatomy and exaggerates the space between the bones for teaching purposes.

However, we can look at real skulls and see the difference between a normal skull and that of an experienced meditator. The pictures of the next two skulls are actual human skulls. Of course, since they are old, they have shrunk and dehydrated over time. The first picture shows the skull of a regular human (fig. 6.6). You can see that the coronal and sagittal sutures are distinct but somewhat filled in, which is an indication of limited range of motion.

The second picture is the skull of a Buddhist lama (teacher) that has been reverently carved and preserved (see fig. 6.7 on page 150). Even

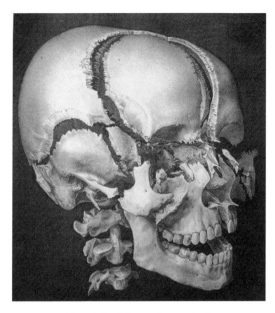

Fig. 6.5. A Beauchene skull

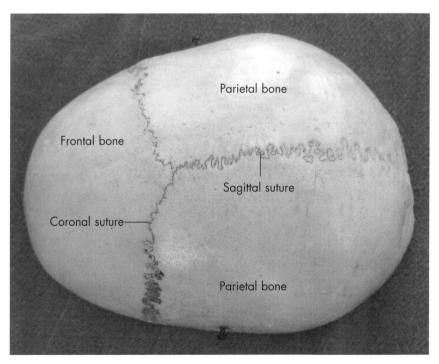

Fig. 6.6. Normal human skull

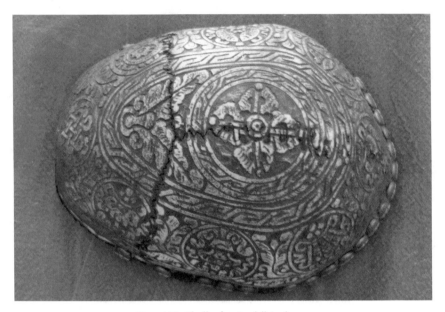

Fig. 6.7. Skull of a Buddhist lama

though it, too, is dehydrated, it is possible to see the significant amount of space along the sutures. Meditative practice opens the sutures, allowing more motility and mobility. The opening also allows more light to penetrate into the skull. If we remember $E=mc^2$, then we understand that more light translates into more energy.

Cranial Flexion and Extension—The Foundations of Craniosacral Work

Cranial movement has two main phases, flexion and extension (figs. 6.8 and 6.9). Flexion is the contraction or inhalation phase. In Chi Kung terms, it would be the yin part of our movements. Extension is the expansion, exhalation, or yang phase. All of the bones of the cranium have this respiratory motion of inhalation and exhalation, contraction and expansion. As measured by scientists, the actual movement of the bones is very small, less than half the thickness of a sheet of paper. However, our internal subjective experience of this wavelike movement may be that it is quite large and even oceanic in feeling.

CRANIAL FLEXION AND EXTENSION

	FLEXION	EXTENSION
Cranium	Widens, shortens	Narrows, lengthens
Cerebrospinal fluid	Fills, pressure rises	Empties, pressure falls
Single bones	Move toward feet	Move toward ears
Paired bones (fig. 6.10)	Rotate out	Rotate in

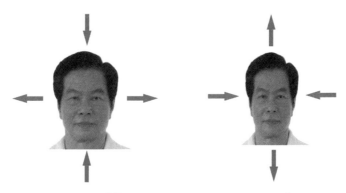

Fig. 6.8. Cranial flexion   Fig. 6.9. Cranial extension

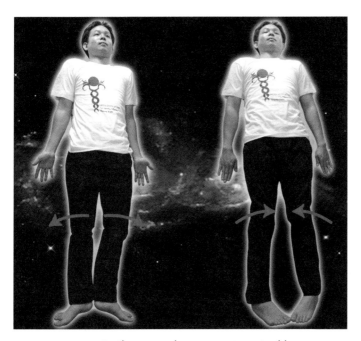

Fig. 6.10. Flexion and extension in paired bones

The motility of the bones—their natural subconscious movement into flexion and extension—tells us a lot about the health of our system. When we tune our radio receiver to the Cranial Wave, we are listening for bone motility. The greater the range and the more balanced the motion of the Cranial Wave, the healthier we are. If the bones and cerebrospinal fluid are blocked, then the chi cannot flow. As Chi Kung practitioners, once we notice the blockages, we can care for ourselves by using our practices to reestablish movement.

 ## Feeling Cranial Motility

This is a simple exercise to build our ability to sense the movement of the cranial bones.

1. Sit or lie comfortably. Gently place your palms over your ears.
2. Soften and relax your hands while you deepen your breath.
3. Sense the widening and narrowing of your head as it moves into flexion and extension.
4. If you think you are noticing the movement of your breathing instead of the movement of your cranial bones, find the rhythmic movement and then hold your breath. If the movement continues and the combined contraction and expansion phases are roughly 4–8 seconds, then you have tuned in to the Cranial Wave.

Sphenoid—The Master Bone of the Cranium

Cranial movement is triggered deep inside the skull by the flexion and extension of the sphenoid bone and its articulation with the occiput. Because the sphenoid is wedged in the middle of the head, it causes all the other bones to shift whenever it moves. It is basically the key to the whole osseous (bony) system.

The sphenoid is located in the center of the head, and consists of two greater wings, two lesser wings, and a body (figs. 6.11 and 6.12). Because of the shape of its wings, the sphenoid is sometimes referred to as the butterfly bone. It is positioned so deeply in the skull that the only parts we can touch from the outside are the greater wings. In Craniosacral Work, the sphenoid bone is considered the master bone of the cranium. One reason it is so important is because the movement of the cranial pump initiates at the sphenobasilar joint (SBJ).

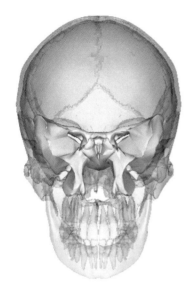

Fig. 6.11. The sphenoid is positioned deep in the center of the head.

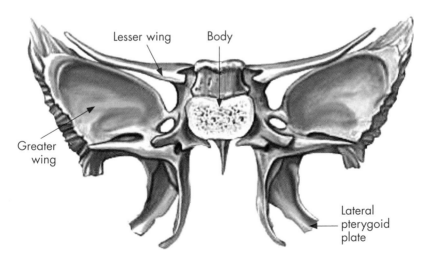

Fig. 6.12. The sphenoid has two greater wings, two lesser wings, and a body. It resembles the shape of a butterfly.

The Sphenobasilar Joint (SBJ)

The sphenoid articulates with the occiput at the sphenobasilar joint (SBJ) (fig. 6.13). When the sphenoid moves into flexion and extension, the movement is transferred to the occiput through the connection of these two bones at the SBJ (figs. 6.14 and 6.15). When the sphenoid is in flexion it nosedives toward the feet. As it does so, a portion of the occiput moves toward the feet as well, causing the angle at the base of the SBJ to get smaller.

The SBJ is considered the most important joint of the cranium: all the bones of the cranium organize and move around this junction. Poetically, the SBJ can be perceived as the center of a flower, with the petals of the sphenoid, temporal bones, and occiput opening out during inhalation and coming toward the center with each exhalation.

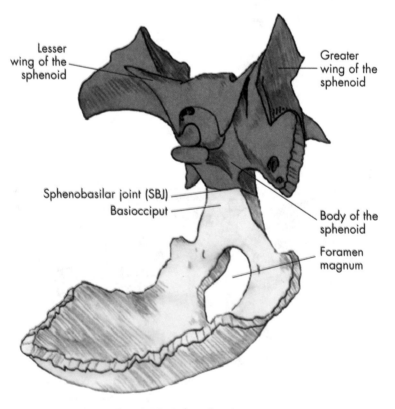

Fig. 6.13. Sphenobasilar joint

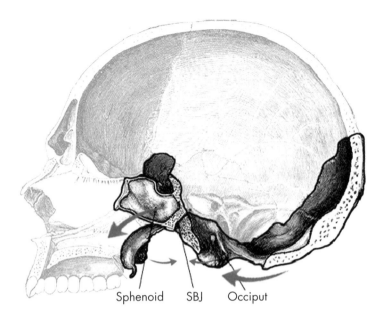

Fig. 6.14. Sphenoid flexion: the sphenoid turns downward and the occiput moves toward the feet. The angle of the SBJ gets smaller.

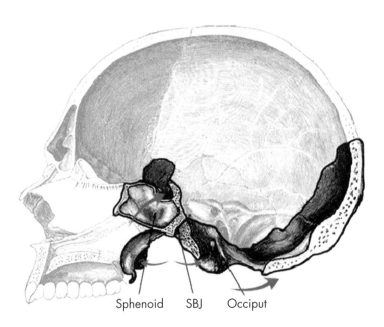

Fig. 6.15. Sphenoid extension: the sphenoid turns upward, the occiput moves toward the sky, and the angle of the SBJ widens.

As the master bone, the sphenoid sets the tone of the entire body. In craniosacral terminology, when the sphenoid is in flexion, all the other bones are said to be in flexion, even though they may be in anatomical extension. Though this convention causes cognitive dissonance for beginning craniosacral students, it is a fundamental principle of Craniosacral Work.

The Sphenoid and Cerebrospinal Fluid

Figure 6.16 shows the foramen magnum—the hole in the occiput through which the medulla oblongata, an extension of the spinal cord, enters and exits the cranium. The dural tube that protects the spinal cord attaches to the foramen magnum, C2, and the sacrum. As the occiput moves, it moves the dural tube, which in turn moves the sacrum and pumps cerebrospinal fluid (fig. 6.17).

This connection from the sphenoid to the occiput via the SBJ, and from the occiput to the sacrum via the dural tube, means that the quality and health of sphenoid movement tends to determine the motility of the pelvis (fig. 6.18).

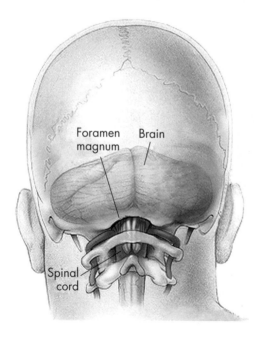

Foramen magnum   Brain

Spinal cord

Fig. 6.16. The gateway between the head and body is the hole in the occiput called the foramen magnum (see also fig. 6.13 on page 154).

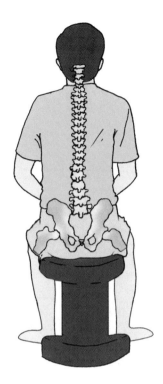

Fig. 6.17. The dura surrounding the spinal cord connects the occiput to the sacrum.

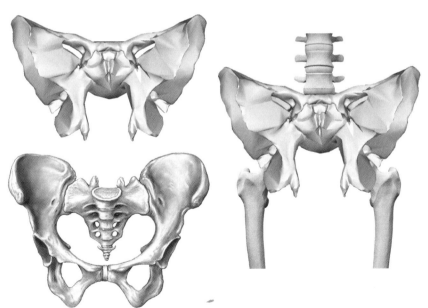

Fig. 6.18. Sphenoid motility affects the sacrum and pelvis.
Note the similarity in shape between the two bones.

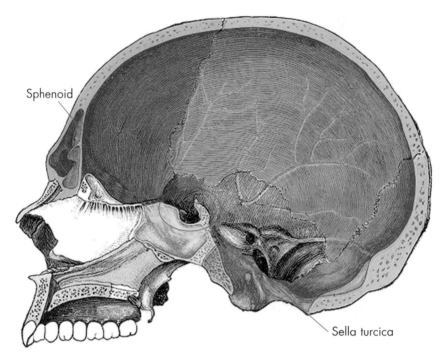

Fig. 6.19. Sphenoid and sella turcica

The Sphenoid and the Pituitary Gland

Another reason the sphenoid is critical to our health, well-being, and spirituality is because of its relationship with the pituitary gland. The pituitary rests in the *sella turcica* (Turkish saddle) portion of the body of the sphenoid (figs. 6.19 and 6.20). The pituitary gland is sometimes called the master gland because, together with the hypothalamus, it regulates the endocrine system and therefore nearly every aspect of our physical body. A fold of tissue called the *diaphragma sellae* roofs the sella turcica with an opening for the pituitary stalk. The gentle wavelike rocking motion of the sphenoid milks the pituitary and stimulates the secretion of the nine hormones that regulate our homeostasis. Thus, anything that affects the sphenoid affects the pituitary, which in turn influences our overall health.

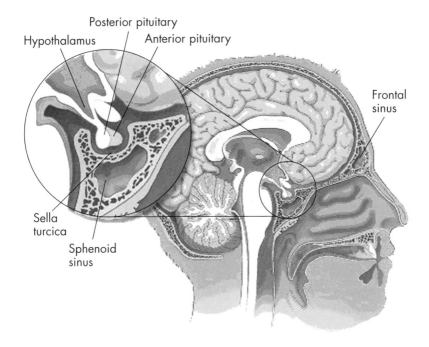

Posterior pituitary
Hypothalamus
Anterior pituitary
Frontal sinus
Sella turcica
Sphenoid sinus

Fig. 6.20. The pituitary sits in the depression formed
by the sella turcica.

The Bone of Light Consciousness

The sphenoid, which forms the back of the eye sockets, is highly sensitive to light and is sometimes called the bone of light consciousness (see fig. 6.21 on page 160). When it is faulted (out of place or restricted in motion), people report experiencing a sense of darkness and depression. They may find themselves thinking of death and notice disturbing dreams. These symptoms frequently occur when the sphenoid is stuck in flexion and does not move well into extension. In flexion, the sphenoid faces downward toward the earth. In extension, it tilts upward toward the light of the spiritual sun and stars. When the sphenoid is able to move freely into extension, we feel buoyant, uplifted, connected, and light.

The sphenoid is also intimately connected with eyesight (see fig. 6.22 on page 160). All but one of the muscles that control eye

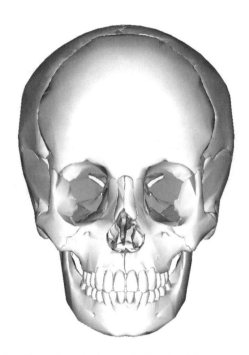

Fig. 6.21. The sphenoid forms the back of the eye sockets.

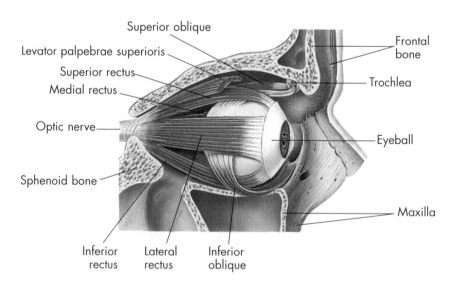

Superior oblique

Levator palpebrae superioris

Superior rectus

Medial rectus

Optic nerve

Sphenoid bone

Frontal bone

Trochlea

Eyeball

Maxilla

Inferior rectus   Lateral rectus   Inferior oblique

Fig. 6.22. The sphenoid affects our vision. All but one of the external muscles that control the eyes attach to the sphenoid or to the tendinous ring that attaches to the sphenoid.

movement attach either directly to the sphenoid or to the tendinous ring that attaches to the wings of the sphenoid. The optic chiasm crosses above the diaphragma sellae just in front of the pituitary.

In the 1990s, Timothy Leary expressed that whoever controls our eyeballs has a strong influence on our thought processes.[2] He was referring to the influence of media, but the comment also highlights the importance of being mindful about our gaze, because our energy follows our attention. We rely on our eyes to bring us information about the world around us. With the advent of computers, many of us spend much of the day staring at a small screen a few feet in front of us. Staying focused at this distance for hours each day is tiring for our eyes, overworking some of our eye muscles and underutilizing others. This situation not only affects our eyes but, as we know now, also affects the internal structures of our cranial bones.

Taoist practices are often very specific about where we should be gazing during the exercises. For example, during the Six Healing Sounds practice, we moved our eyes left and right to delete the negative programing in each organ: the direction of our gaze triggers different muscles to move the sphenoid, activate the cranial pump, and stimulate the pituitary gland. Taoists also alternate opening the eyes wide and squeezing them closed during practice to activate different parts of the brain. When we squeeze our eyes, we connect with the center of the head and activate it. When we release, the chi circulates and flows through the area.

 ## Following the Clock

To help relax the tension in our eyes and balance our eye muscles, we can use the following exercises.

1. Sit comfortably with the spine aligned and relaxed.
2. With your eyes open, imagine that you are looking at the face of an old-fashioned analog clock.

3. Bring your gaze to 12 o'clock. Very slowly begin to move your eyes in a clockwise direction, moving from number to number around the clock.

4. Notice if your eyes want to skip over a number or section of the clock. If they do, spend a few moments moving your eyes back and forth through that area. Invite the movement to be smooth and steady.

5. Make 9 circuits of the clock, then reverse and do 9 circuits in a counterclockwise direction. Pause and spend time in the areas where the movement is jerky or the muscles feel tense. You may notice quite a difference in the quality of movement when you change directions.

6. When you're done, squeeze your eyes closed tightly and then release. Do this 9 times. Feel the increased circulation in your brain and head.

7. Rub your hands together briskly to generate warmth.

8. Place your palms over your eyes and absorb the chi deep into your eye sockets.

9. Notice how your eyes feel different.

You can also do this exercise with your eyes closed, which will allow you to focus more on your sensations. Some people may find it more challenging to go fully around the clock without external visual references.

Energetics of the Craniosacral Bones

The practices in this book can cause physical shifts in the cranium: the sutures may open, the structure of the bones may change, and the shape of the head may shift as well. As we know, physical shifts often then lead to emotional, mental, and energetic shifts. In our practice, it is helpful to know a little more about the energetics of the key bones so that we can better accommodate and encourage their shifts. In his book *The Heart of Listening,* Hugh Milne discusses the following correlations between the bones and their energetics.[3]

Sphenoid

The sphenoid is the seat of the inner eye and relates to our perceptive capacities, clarity, insight, clairvoyance, and dreams (fig. 6.23). The sphenoid is the windshield through which we see ourselves, others, and the world.[4] When it is not in balance, we may feel despairing, depressed, and dark. When the sphenoid moves freely, we are buoyant and filled with an inner light that connects us with Source.

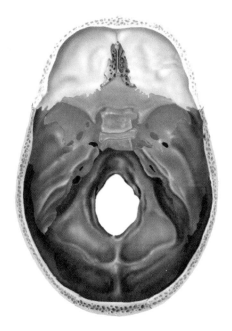

Fig. 6.23. The sphenoid—seat of the inner eye

Occiput

The occiput is the base of the skull—the part of the head that rests on the floor when we lie down (see fig. 6.24 on page 164). It is a tall bone that actually reaches as high as the level of our eyes. The occiput is connected with power, authority, and being in charge. It is also the beginning of the channel of our inner eye. When the occiput is out of alignment, we may experience feelings of betrayal or have difficulty trusting others.

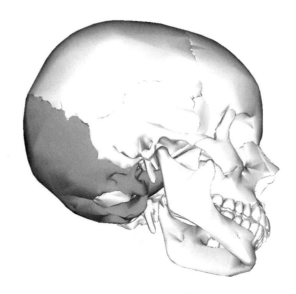

Fig. 6.24. Occipital bone

The medulla oblongata, which becomes the brain stem, passes through the foramen magnum of the occiput. In addition, 95 percent of venous blood exits the head through the occiput's jugular foramen. People often experience a sense of pressure or congestion in the head when energy rises and gets stuck there. When we reduce restrictions in the occiput, energy can flow downward, releasing that pressure.

Frontal

The frontal bone is what we generally think of as the forehead (fig. 6.25). The energetics of the frontal bone involve both stubborn determination and wisdom. In its highest aspect, the frontal bone helps us choose wisely rather than letting raw instinct or emotions drive our behavior. The channel of the inner eye exits through this bone in the area between our eyebrows—often called the third eye. The frontal bone is designed to protect the brain and withstand strong forces, so it rarely faults even under significant pressure. When it is in balance, we are in touch with our highest ethics, our cognition is sharp, and we can access our intuition clearly via the third eye.

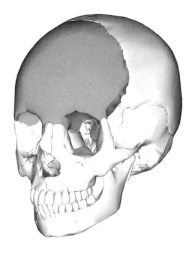

Fig. 6.25. Frontal bone

Parietals

The two parietal bones are found on the sides and top of the head (fig. 6.26). They are home to the crown soul. When the parietals are open, we feel deeply connected to the cosmos. This feeling of opening has been described as the blooming of the thousand-petalled lotus. When the parietals are constricted, we may have a difficult time getting in touch with divinity. In contrast, as the parietals and crown center open, we often experience a sense of transcendence and oneness with All that Is.

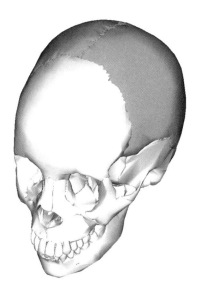

Fig. 6.26. Parietal bones

Temporals

The two temporal bones are in the region of the ears (fig. 6.27). They are connected to our physical and metaphorical balance, our sense of time, and our flexibility in life. When the temporals are faulted, we may experience hearing issues, tinnitus, nausea, difficulty in gauging time, and a lack of balance. On the other hand, when the temporals are communicating well with each other and are able to move smoothly into both flexion and extension, we are able to digest new experiences, maintain our equanimity in the face of challenges, and easily balance our inner and outer lives.

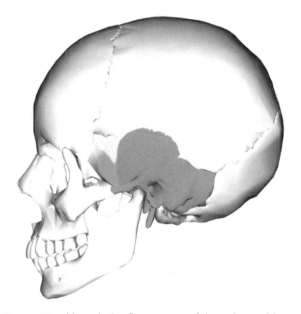

Fig. 6.27. Although the flat portion of the sphenoid bone just behind our eye sockets is often called the temple, it should not be confused with the temporal bone, which sits behind the sphenoid in the area of the ear.

Maxillae

The two maxillae form the upper jaw (fig. 6.28). They are related to our ability to speak our truth, to our sense of loyalty, and to our capacity to either defend ourselves or attack when encountering aggression.

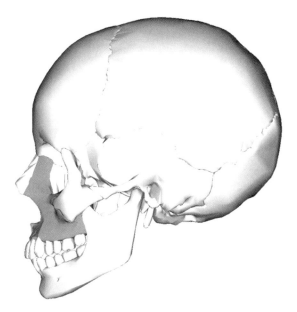

Fig. 6.28. Maxillary bones

Both the maxillae and mandible are strongly affected by dental and orthodontic work. When out of sync, we may experience headaches, sinusitis, and visual problems. When our maxillae are aligned and free to move, we are able to communicate smoothly and clearly, express affection easily, and see projects through to completion.

Mandible

The mandible, our lower jaw, holds the energy of our identity (see fig. 6.29 on page 168). As part of the throat soul, it can express aggression, tenacity, sensuality, and sexuality: we grit our teeth, set our jaws, enjoy food, and sing love songs with our mouths. Stress causes many of us to hold tension in the mandible, which may reflect the repression of emotions or things we are not willing to express. Such tension can also lead to temporomandibular joint (TMJ) pain.

The mandible is closely associated with the neck, where the center of mass for the 136 muscles involved in chewing, swallowing, and speaking is located at the second cervical vertebra. The neck is also the

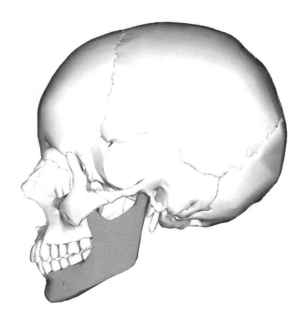

Fig. 6.29. Mandible

source of mandibular movement. This relationship means that the neck and lower jaw have a strong effect on each other: neck pain is often related to clenching of the jaw or grinding of the teeth, and mandibular pain may be the result of chronic neck tension. On an energetic level, freeing the mandible allows us to express who we are more fully and authentically and also helps us turn our heads to view the world from a new perspective.

Sacrum

The sacrum is our root and connection to the earth (fig. 6.30). It holds the energies of security, safety, stability, sexuality, support, and spirituality. The origin of the word *sacrum* is *sacer,* which means "sacred" in Latin. This bone is considered the beginning of the path to enlightenment, which ascends the spine to the crown. When the sacrum is out of balance, we may feel insecure and unstable. We may have difficulty knowing where we stand or what we stand for in life. However, when we are connected with the sacrum, we feel supported, grounded, and on our path.

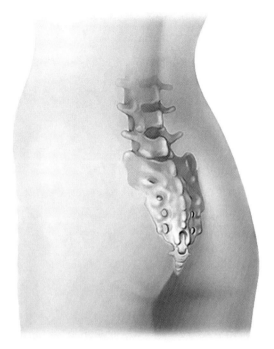

Fig. 6.30. Sacrum

The sacrum regulates the bones and bone marrow. If we want to stimulate and strengthen the bones, we can reach all of them by working with the sacrum because it is the physical and energetic cornerstone of our structure.

Connecting with Our Bones

Since we may not have much experience with the energy of our bones and their deep wisdom, it can be useful to spend time connecting with them.

 ## Bone Breathing

1. Sit comfortably on the edge of your chair with your feet flat, about shoulder-width apart.
2. Feel the soles of your feet breathing. Feel your eight sacral holes breathing. Feel the bone marrow in your sacrum breathing.

3. As you inhale, connect your feet with the earth and draw earth energy upward to your sacrum.

4. With each exhalation, imagine you are squeezing and twisting your bones as if you were wringing out a wet towel. Squeeze out any waste or toxins from deep inside your sacrum. Feel the space that is created.

5. On your inhalation, sense earth energy welling up through the Bubbling Springs point on the bottom of your feet.

6. On your exhalation, invite the chi to expand into the space that has opened up and fill the sacral foramen. When the foramen are full, feel the abundance of the earth nourish and rejuvenate the bone marrow deep inside your bones.

Cranial Bone Sensing

Ancient Taoists could hear the wisdom of the rocks and mountains. Just because rocks move so slowly that the movement is almost imperceptible does not mean that movement does not exist. By cultivating our ability to listen to the quiet deep voice of our bones (our internal structure), we build our capacity to listen to the Earth's structure as well.

1. Begin by sitting comfortably with your head over your heart and your head and heart over your sacrum. Allow your breath to be slow and smooth. Feel the rhythmic expansion and contraction of your lungs.

2. Turn your awareness to your head. Feel your head breathing from deep inside, getting shorter and wider, then lengthening and narrowing.

3. Bring your hands to the base of your skull at your occiput. Connect in with its power. Feel the occiput resting against your hand and relax into the support. Find the depression at the bottom of the bone: your sacrum connects to the occiput through the dura in this area. Draw earth energy up from the sacrum through to the occiput. Press your fingers gently inward and upward in the direc-

tion of the mid-eyebrow point. Invite the channel of your inner eye to open.

4. When you are ready, bring your hands to the frontal bone, which houses the exit point of the inner eye. When we are grounded and stabilized with the earth energy of the sacrum and the power of the occiput, it is easier to open our perceptions to the heavens. Feel the wisdom of the inner eye balance and uplift both your stubborn determination and your analytical, rational thought processes.

5. At the right time, bring your hands to the temporal bones around your ears. Feel the temporals breathing, balancing left and right, yin and yang with every inhalation and exhalation. Drop deeper into the quality of balance; balance in your physical body, balance in your emotions, balance in life. From this place of balance, you can open to hear more of the world around you, and also to hear more of what your inner guidance and the Tao have to share with you. As you rest here, you may feel a sense of timelessness and equanimity.

6. Next, bring your hands to your lower jaw to connect with the mandible. Move your jaw slightly forward and feel its strength, tenacity, and yang nature. Relax your jaw and move your tongue around the inside of your mouth; tune in to the mandible's capacity for sensuality and sexuality. Our teeth are bones too: tap your teeth together lightly. Feel the vibration move through your mandible, awakening your throat soul and connecting with the ability to express yourself clearly and authentically.

7. Feel your upper jaw, the maxillae. Tap your teeth together again and feel the upper jaw activating. Move your lips back to bare your teeth and feel your ability to take action to defend and protect yourself when necessary and appropriate. Relax your upper jaw into a smile. With this smile, let it express the inner truth of who you are. Press your tongue to the roof of your mouth.

8. Let the vibration of your smile rise upward until it reaches the sphenoid. Bring your hands to the sides of your head to touch the greater wings of this butterfly bone in the flat area just behind your

eye sockets. Allow your awareness to follow the wings into the center of the skull. Feel the light of your smile resonate with this bone of light consciousness. Notice the inner light filling your cranium. Allow that light to bring clarity to your perceptive abilities and offer insights.

9. Move your hands to the top and sides of your head, the location of your parietal bones. As the parietal bones soften, the crown opens and light from above connects with the light from within; they become one. Feel your smile grow as it absorbs this spiritual light. Receive the cosmic download and rest in Oneness.

10. Invite your smile and the sense of oneness down to your heart. Let the heart and its powerful electromagnetic field radiate light, love, and oneness out to the rest of your body.

11. When your body is full, allow the rest of the energy to move down to your tan tien.

12. Spiral the energy in 9 times and seal it into your tan tien.

CONNECTING ALL THE PARTS
TO FEEL ENERGY FLOW

Taoism emphasizes the importance having awareness of both the parts and the whole. Having looked at our pumps, organs, and tan tiens, and having increased the Flow in our physical, mental, and emotional bodies, we can now broaden our focus to the whole energy body and increase the flow of our chi.

The exercises below will help you to feel the connections between your bones and your pumps, your tan tiens and your organs, your mass and your energy.

Riding the Horse

1. Begin by sitting comfortably on a chair with your feet flat against the floor and your spine aligned with your head over your heart

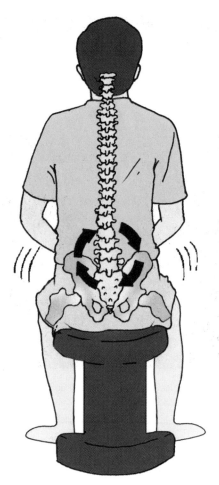

Fig. 6.31. Riding the Horse

over your hips. Rock your spine from the sitting bones back and forth as if you are riding a horse (fig. 6.31). Activate all the vertebrae of the spine up to your head and awaken the nerves.

Swimming Dragon

1. Imagine you are a powerful and fluid dragon swimming in a private ocean in your upper tan tien/heaven (the cerebrospinal fluid in your head).

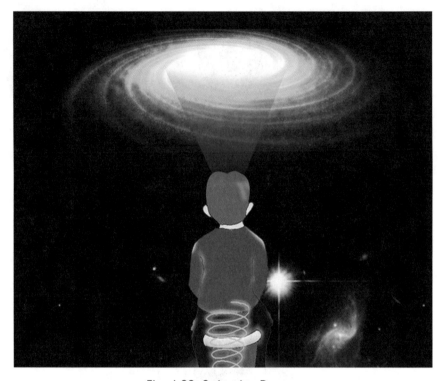

Fig. 6.32. Swimming Dragon

2. You want to visit earth (the lower tan tien at your sacrum), and know that the easiest path is to swim down the spine.
3. Feel the swimming dragon descending your spine until it reaches the lower tan tien (fig. 6.32).

Fire Dragon

The Fire Dragon lives deep in the sea. He lives so deep that his tail sometimes comes in contact with the Fire under the Sea—the molten magma that lies underneath the earth's crust.

1. Imagine you are a strong and active dragon swimming in the deep ocean currents. Your tail touches the molten lava and sends a jolt of energy up your tail to your head (fig. 6.33).

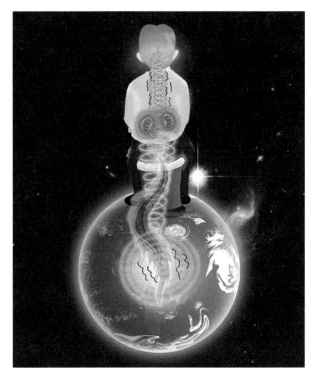

Fig. 6.33. Fire Dragon

2. As the spark travels from the tip of your coccyx through all the bones of your spine to the occiput, the charge may be so strong that you jump.
3. Feel the chi energizing and charging your bones.

Microcosmic Orbit

The Microcosmic Orbit connects us to the universe within ourselves, bringing us to a state of unity and internal oneness. We can view the Microcosmic Orbit as the natural movement of water in nature. The powerful sun shines on the water (kidneys). The light descends into the depths of the water, heating it up. The steam ascends up the mountain (the spine) and as it rises, it cools. Once it reaches the peak of the mountain (the crown), it begins to condense into a mist, which flows downward until it reaches the Sea of Chi, completing the circuit.

With the Microcosmic Orbit meditation, we open our awareness to the whole body and whole energy field (fig. 6.34). This larger flow is called the Fluid Tide; connecting with its deeper flow enables us to access more power and more health.

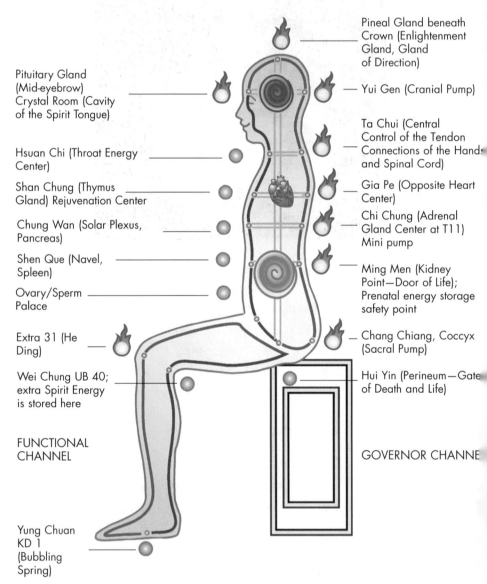

Pineal Gland beneath Crown (Enlightenment Gland, Gland of Direction)

Pituitary Gland (Mid-eyebrow) Crystal Room (Cavity of the Spirit Tongue)

Yui Gen (Cranial Pump)

Ta Chui (Central Control of the Tendon Connections of the Hands and Spinal Cord)

Hsuan Chi (Throat Energy Center)

Shan Chung (Thymus Gland) Rejuvenation Center

Gia Pe (Opposite Heart Center)

Chung Wan (Solar Plexus, Pancreas)

Chi Chung (Adrenal Gland Center at T11) Mini pump

Shen Que (Navel, Spleen)

Ovary/Sperm Palace

Ming Men (Kidney Point—Door of Life); Prenatal energy storage safety point

Extra 31 (He Ding)

Chang Chiang, Coccyx (Sacral Pump)

Wei Chung UB 40; extra Spirit Energy is stored here

Hui Yin (Perineum—Gate of Death and Life)

FUNCTIONAL CHANNEL

GOVERNOR CHANNEL

Yung Chuan KD 1 (Bubbling Spring)

Fig. 6.34. Microcosmic Orbit

1. Sit comfortably with your feet flat against the floor and your spine aligned with your head over heart over hips. Press the tip of your tongue against your upper palate.
2. Turn your senses inward and bring your mind to the lower tan tien.
3. Focus on the lower tan tien, where Original Chi resides, in the area between the navel, kidneys, and sexual organs.
4. Take 9 or 18 deep breaths in and out, then smile to your tan tien.
5. With your mind and eyes, gather and spiral the energy in your tan tien into a chi ball.
6. Spiral the chi ball down to your sexual center (the Ovarian or Sperm Palace).
7. Move the chi ball down to the perineum and down to the soles of the feet (Yung Chuan).
8. Invite the energy up from the bottom of the feet to the perineum (Hui Yin) and the sacrum/coccyx (Chang Chiang).
9. From the sacrum, the energy rises to the Door of Life, on the spine directly behind the navel.
10. Feel the energy rising to the midpoint of the spine—T11/Chi Chung, the point opposite the solar plexus.
11. The energy continues to rise to Gia Pe, the point opposite the heart.
12. Draw the energy up to Yu Zhen (Jade Pillow) at the base of the skull.
13. From there the energy ascends to the crown point/Bai Hui and the pineal gland.
14. Next, move the energy ball downward to Yin Tang and the pituitary at the mid-eyebrow point.
15. The energy flows downward through the palate and tongue to the throat at Hsuan Chi.
16. From the throat, energy descends to the heart center at Shan Chung.
17. From the heart, it moves to the solar plexus/Chung Wan.
18. The energy then descends to the navel/Shen Que.
19. Circulate energy through the Microcosmic Orbit at least 9 times.

As the energy begins to move more and more smoothly, become aware of the Flow through the entire circuit: the orbit connects all the different parts of us. Notice that it begins to move on its own without your needing to consciously direct it.

20. After a while, you may feel chi flowing through you like a tide with a rhythm of its own. You may also feel a wave of energy flowing through the whole channel, lighting up the entire orbit at once. Notice the feeling of integration and wholeness.

21. To close, allow the energy to slow down and gather at your navel.

Men: cover your navel with your right hand, and place your left hand on top of the right. Spiral the energy outward 36 times in a clockwise direction, then inward 24 times in a counterclockwise direction.

Women: cover your navel with your left hand, and place your right hand over the left. Spiral the energy outward 36 times in a counterclockwise direction, then inward 24 times in a clockwise direction.

Note: Pay attention to the Flow all along the orbit. At first, it is natural to notice areas where the energy disappears or does not seem to flow as smoothly. Some people may have difficulty feeling energy flowing through the orbit at all. In these cases, spend more time doing rapid Bellows Breathing or Spinal Cord Breathing before beginning your Microcosmic Orbit practice. This will increase the flow of chi so that it is easier to notice and so that it has more "volume" as it moves through the entire circuit.

MERIDIAN FLOW

No discussion of Taoist energy flows would be complete without mentioning the meridians, the energy pathways or channels through which chi energy flows. In Chinese medicine, the twelve regular meridians correspond with and connect to our internal organs. Like the tides, energy ebbs and flows along these pathways. Each of the twelve meridians reaches its peak potency for two hours each day, making a twenty-four-hour cycle (see fig. 6.35 on page 180).

The chart below provides more detail on the two-hour period when each meridian is activated and dominant. The process of shifting from one meridian to another is automatic and continuous. During the day, as the energies of the meridians shift, our moods, thoughts, and physical functions may fluctuate as well.

MERIDIAN BODY CLOCK

ORGAN	TIME	ACTION
Lung	3–5 a.m.	Respiratory system, skin, immune system
Large Intestine	5–7 a.m.	Elimination of solid waste, removal of toxins, letting go
Stomach	7–9 a.m.	Digestion of food, ability to take in resources
Spleen	9–11 a.m.	Blood sugar regulation, chi distribution
Heart	11 a.m.–1 p.m.	Cardiac system, circulation, memory, communication; governs mind and emotions
Small Intestine	1–3 p.m.	Assimilation of nutrients, absorption of water, sorting/integration of ideas
Bladder	3–5 p.m.	Elimination of fluid wastes, flexibility and armoring
Kidney	5–7 p.m.	Bones, adrenals, stamina
Pericardium	7–9 p.m.	Protects heart, balances emotions, integrates heart/mind
Tripler Warmer	9–11 p.m.	Body balance, relationships, endocrine system, autonomic nervous system, appetites
Gall Bladder	11 p.m.–1 a.m.	Breakdown of fats; governs judgment and planning
Liver	1–3 a.m.	Digestion of fats; governs eyes, nervous system, detoxification, adaptability, growth, decision making

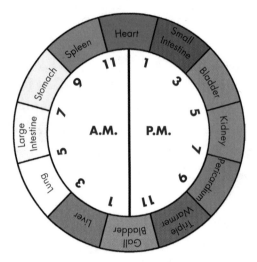

Fig. 6.35. Meridian Body Clock

 Brushing the Yin and Yang Meridians

If you are unfamiliar with the meridians or would like a simple easy way to get the meridians flowing, use this quick exercise, which traces the yin and yang meridians of the arms, legs, and trunk (fig. 6.36).

The three arm yin meridians (Heart, Pericardium, and Lung) start on the upper chest and flow to the fingers. The three leg yin meridians (Kidney, Spleen, and Liver) start at the feet and flow up to the torso. The arm yang meridians (Large Intestine, Small Intestine, and Triple Warmer) start at the fingers and flow through the arms to the head. The leg yang meridians (Bladder, Gall Bladder, and Stomach) start on the head and flow down through the torso to the toes.

If you would like to trace each meridian separately in the order of the body clock, use the more detailed variation that follows this exercise.

1. Sit or stand comfortably and spend a moment to bring your awareness inside.
2. Notice how you are in the moment, so you can feel the difference after you have opened the meridians.
3. Begin by doing 9 rounds of abdominal breathing and 9 rounds of reverse breathing.

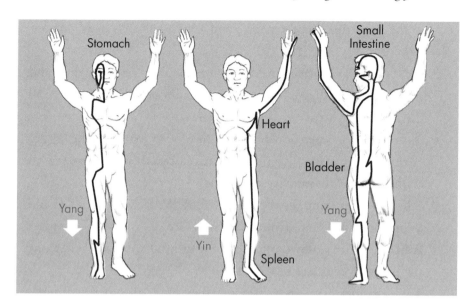

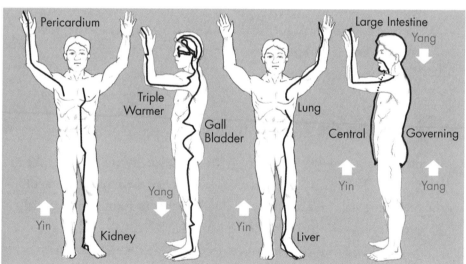

Fig. 6.36. Organ meridians

4. Hold your hands out to the sides, palms up to gather chi.
5. Clap your hands together and rub them briskly.
6. On your next inhalation, use the palm of your right hand to brush up the inside of your left arm, from fingertips to shoulder.
7. Exhale and brush down the back of the left arm from the shoulder

to the fingertips. Repeat steps 6 and 7 with your left hand on your right arm.

8. Bend down and place your hands on the inside of your feet and ankles. As you inhale, brush up the insides of your feet, legs, and thighs to your hips.

9. As you exhale, sweep down the outside of your legs from the hips to knees, then all the way to the outer edge of your feet and toes. This connects with the yang leg meridians.

10. Inhale and brush up the top of your foot, the front of your legs and thighs, and the front of your chest and face.

11. Exhale and brush down the back of your head and back, and along the backs of your legs to the heels.

12. Trace the meridian circuit 3 times, then guide the energy to settle into the tan tien.

13. Feel the energy of the meridians flowing freely and gathering in the tan tien. Seal it with 9 circles.

14. Notice what has changed.

Tracing the Meridian Flow

In this exercise you will brush down the meridians in the order of the body clock. Note that each meridian starts near the ending point of the preceding one, and that they all link together to form a full circuit. Refer to figures 6.37–6.43 to see the pathways.

You will be using your intention to connect with each channel, so there is no need to be concerned about specific points. However, learning the pathways in more detail will enable you to understand and connect with them on an even deeper level.

1. Sit or stand comfortably and spend a moment to bring your awareness inside.

2. Notice how you are in the moment, so you can see the difference after you have opened the meridians.

3. Begin by doing 9 rounds of abdominal breathing and 9 rounds of reverse breathing.

4. Hold your hands out to the sides, palms up to gather the chi.

5. Clap your hands together and rub them briskly, then begin to trace the meridians as detailed below.

6. **Lung:** Start on the left side of your chest just in front of your shoulder. With your right hand, brush down the palm side of your arm to the thumb tip. Connect with the Lungs and your respiratory system. Feel your immune system coming online. Repeat on the opposite side.

7. **Large Intestine:** The Large Intestine meridian starts nearby at the tip of your index finger. Use your right hand to brush up the back of the left arm from the index finger to your neck to the corner of your left nostril. Connect with the Large Intestine. Let go of anything you are ready to release. Repeat on the opposite side.

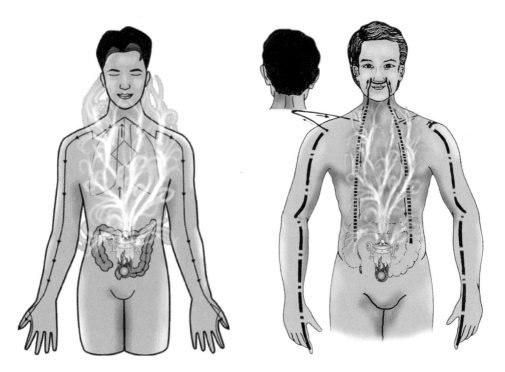

Fig. 6.37. Lung and Large Intestine meridians

8. **Stomach:** Bring both hands to touch the cheekbones underneath the eyes. Sweep down to the jaw, follow the jaw to its angle, up to the forehead to the hairline, then down to the throat, front of the chest, abdomen, and front of the thighs. Move laterally to the outside of the knee and follow the lateral edge of the femur to the ankle and all the way to the lateral edge of the second toe. Bring your awareness to the Stomach and its ability to take in nourishment.

9. **Spleen:** Start at the inside corner of the big toes. Brush up the inside of the ankle, leg, and inner thigh, through the hip crease to the outer edge of the torso. Continue up the outer front edge of the torso to the chest, then back down to the ribs in front of the armpit. Focus on the Spleen and feel the chi being distributed throughout the body.

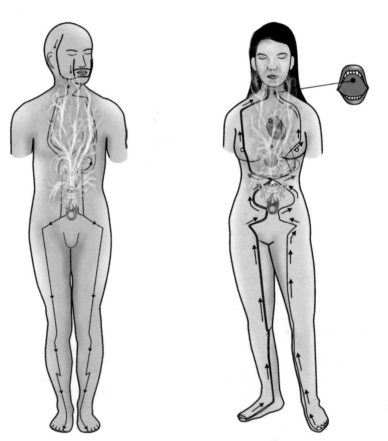

Fig. 6.38. Stomach and Spleen meridians

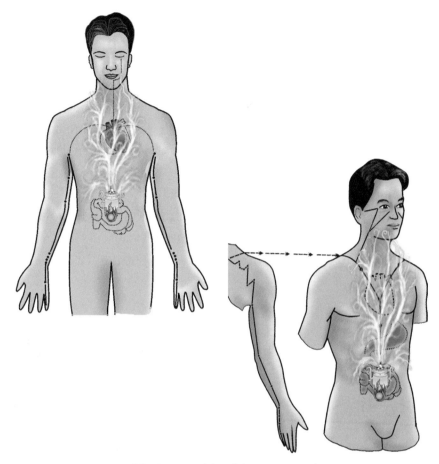

Fig. 6.39. Heart and Small Intestine meridians

10. **Heart:** Bring your right hand to your left armpit and brush down the palm side of the arm to the inside tip of the little finger. Touch into the energy of the Heart with its capacity to communicate and lead. Repeat on the right side with your left hand.

11. **Small Intestine:** Use your right hand to brush up the back of your left arm from the outside tip of the little finger to the scapula. Continue on to the neck, the left cheekbone, and backward toward the front of the left ear. Connect with the energy of the Small Intestine and its ability to take things in and sort them. Repeat on the opposite side.

12. **Urinary Bladder:** Begin with both hands at the inner corner of the eyes and move up along the forehead, over the top of the head, and down the neck. On the back, the meridian splits into four branches (two on each side of the spine), which run down the back parallel and lateral to the spine. All four branches continue down the buttocks and back of the legs to the knee. The meridians rejoin behind the knee and flow down the calf to the outside of the ankle, ending at the outside corner of the little toe. Tune in to the Bladder and its ability to flush out toxins and bring fluidity to life.

13. **Kidney:** Start at the soles of the feet and brush up the insides of the ankles and thighs, across the pelvis and abdomen. Continue up the front of the chest to the bottom inside corner of the collarbone. Connect to the energy of the Kidneys, which affects our bones, adrenal system, and overall stamina.

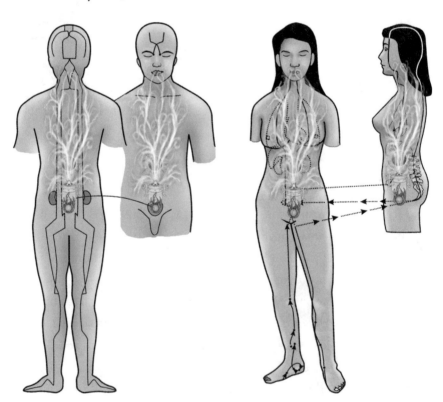

Fig. 6.40. Urinary Bladder and Kidney meridians

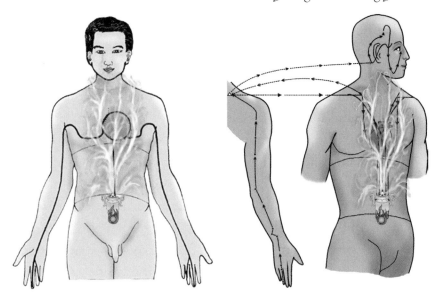

Fig. 6.41. Pericardium and Triple Warmer meridians

14. **Pericardium:** Use your right hand to span your left collarbone. Find the midway point of the collarbone and move directly downward into the fourth space in between the ribs below the collarbone. Now move one finger's width to the outside and that is where the Pericardium meridian starts. Brush your right hand from that point up onto the front of your left shoulder and then down along the inner aspect of the left arm, through the palm to the tip of the middle finger. Focus on the energy of the Pericardium. Sense its ability to protect the Heart as well as integrate the Heart and Mind. Repeat on the right side with your left hand.

15. **Triple Warmer:** Turn the left hand palm down and use the right hand to trace the Triple Warmer meridian. Beginning on the outer tip of the ring finger, brush up the back of the left hand and arm to the back of the left shoulder and side of the neck. Continue, moving behind the ear to the outside edge of the left eyebrow. Tune in to the Triple Warmer, which connects the three tan tiens. Feel the body, emotions, and mind coming into balance and our relationships coming into harmony. Repeat on the right side with your left hand.

16. **Gall Bladder:** Using both hands, trace each side of the Gall Bladder meridian by starting at the outer corner of the eyes, moving back toward the ears, forward to the temples, and back to the base of the skull on each side. From there ascend the side of the skull to the forehead above the eyes, back up over the top of the head, along the neck, across the front of the shoulders, and down the sides of the body and legs to the fourth toe. Sense the Gall Bladder energy and its strength in planning and execution.

17. **Liver:** With both hands, start at the lateral side of each big toe and brush up the top of the foot, the inside of the lower leg, knee, and thigh. Continue along the inside of the groin to the outside of the waist, then forward onto the ribcage. Feel the Liver energy with its ability to adapt, change, and grow.

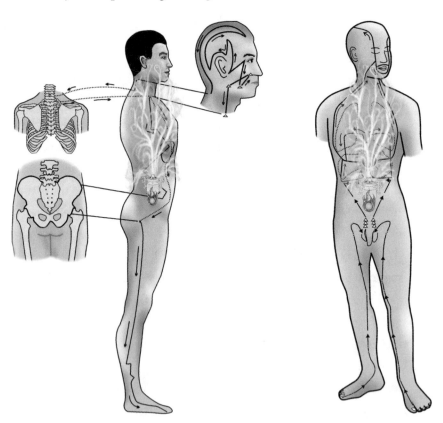

Fig. 6.42. Gall Bladder and Liver meridians

18. **Lung:** Connect with the nearby Lung meridian on the chest and repeat step 6 above, brushing down to the thumbs on both sides to complete the meridian body clock circuit.

19. Feel the energy flowing from one meridian to the other creating a complete and continuous circuit (fig. 6.43).

20. Notice what has changed since the beginning of this exercise.

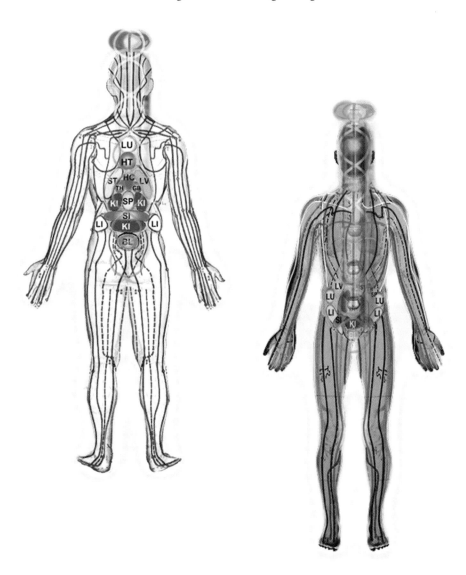

Fig. 6.43. Meridian pathways

Like the bones, each meridian has its own gifts and wisdom. Spending time meditating with and listening to each meridian, and tuning in to the unique flow of each one, deepens our practice and our connection with the entire energy system.

Note: If you have a bamboo or metal beater, then you can also do Bone Marrow Chi Kung to activate the meridians.

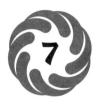

Becoming Liquid Light

The Endocrine System and Spiritual Practice

Now that we have a solid foundation with and connection to the energetics and wisdom of our bones and channels, we can turn our attention to the other key influencers of energy flow and spiritual growth. By deepening our understanding of cranial structures, neurochemistry, and subtle rhythmic energetic movements we can gain insight into the famous Crystal Palace, crucial for spiritual awakening, that is mentioned in many wisdom teachings.

BIOLOGICAL FUNCTIONS OF THE ENDOCRINE SYSTEM

In both Craniosacral Work and Taoist practice, the endocrine system is a critical gateway joining physical function with spiritual experience. The endocrine system includes the following glands: the pituitary, pineal, hypothalamus, thyroid, parathyroid, adrenals, pancreas, and ovaries/testes. These glands use hormones (rather than the electrical impulses used by the nervous system) to effect changes in our body, emotions, cognition, and energy. Hormones are chemical messengers that circulate through the body via the bloodstream and coordinate critical body functions. They increase or reduce nerve impulses and can also act as neurotransmitters.

The hypothalamus, pituitary, and pineal glands play particularly important roles in spiritual experience and will be explored in greater detail in the sections that follow (fig. 7.1).

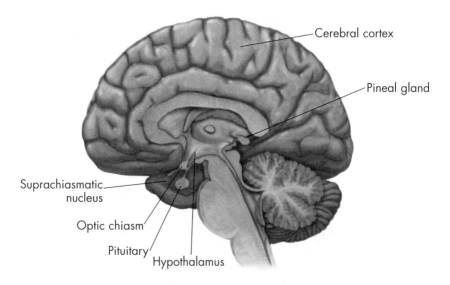

Fig. 7.1. The pineal, pituitary, and hypothalamus glands reside deep in the brain.

The Hypothalamus/Pituitary Relationship

With access to both the nervous and endocrine systems, the hypothalamus plays a central role in linking the two. It is also connected with the limbic system, a center for our feelings and emotions. When entrained with the pituitary gland, the hypothalamus therefore has the ability to affect most of the major systems and organ functions in the body as well as our emotions. Together, the hypothalamus and pituitary regulate all of our basic survival processes including body temperature, hunger, thirst, fatigue, growth, sleep, weight, sexual function, pain relief, blood pressure, circadian rhythms, and stress responses such as fight or flight.

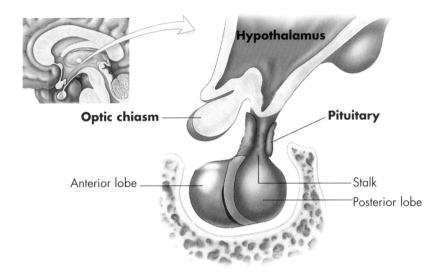

Fig. 7.2. Location of the hypothalamus and pituitary

The hypothalamus is about the size of an almond and is located just behind the optic chiasm (fig. 7.2). It secretes neurohormones that communicate with the pituitary gland, signaling the release or inhibition of key pituitary hormones.

The pituitary gland has two major lobes, which are distinctly different embryologically, anatomically, and functionally. Altogether, the pituitary is about the size of a pea; it sits below the hypothalamus, cradled in the sella turcica of the sphenoid bone. Because the pituitary is enclosed by the sphenoid, it is highly sensitive to misalignments or restrictions in the movement of that bone. If you press your tongue to the roof of your mouth at the soft palate, you are pressing on the underside of the pituitary.

The hypothalamus communicates with the anterior lobe of the pituitary via blood vessels, and connects directly with the posterior lobe through the pituitary stalk or infundibulum. Although the pituitary gland has often been referred to as the master gland because it appears to control the endocrine system, the hypothalamus plays a more crucial role in this system than previously thought. The hypothalamus receives and integrates information from the rest of the body and then secretes the neurohormones that release or inhibit key pituitary hormones. By signaling and directing the pituitary, the hypothalamus plays a critical part in the endocrine system.

Functions of the Pituitary

The anterior lobe of the pituitary secretes seven key hormones that are related to lactation, the release of testosterone, and the production of sex, thyroid, and human growth hormones. The posterior lobe does not produce hormones, but stores and releases two important ones made in the brain: oxytocin and vasopressin. Oxytocin fosters maternal instincts, bonding between mates, trust, and sexual pleasure. Vasopressin influences circadian rhythms, the reabsorption of water into the bloodstream, and also stimulates paternal protective and caring instincts.

The pituitary relates to our growth. When it begins to vibrate in synchrony with the pineal gland, we are inspired to grow and renew ourselves both physically and spiritually.

PITUITARY HORMONES

ANTERIOR LOBE OF PITUITARY		
Hormone	**Target**	**Action**
Adrenocorticotropic hormone (ACTH)	Adrenal gland	Secretes glucocorticoids (cortisol), mineralocorticoids, and androgens (male sex hormones)
Thyroid-stimulating hormone (TSH)	Thyroid gland	Secretes thyroid hormones
Follicle-stimulating hormone (FSH)	Gonads	Stimulates growth of reproductive system, estrogens, production of sperm
Luteinizing hormone (LH)	Gonads	Affects progesterone, testosterone, and ovulation
Growth hormone (GH)	Liver, adipose tissue	Promotes growth
Prolactin (PRL)	Ovaries, mammary glands	Secretes estrogen and progesterone, stimulates milk production
Melanin-stimulating hormone (MSH) (Intermediate Lobe)	Brain	Secretes melanin, increases skin pigmentation, influences appetite and sexual arousal

PITUITARY HORMONES (CONT.)

POSTERIOR LOBE OF PITUITARY		
Hormone	Target	Action
Vasopressin/antidiuretic hormone (ADH)	Kidneys, brain	Influences water retention, blood vessel constriction, and paternal instincts
Oxytocin	Uterus, mammary glands	Influences pair bonding, maternal instincts, sexual pleasure

The Pineal Gland

The pineal is located in the center of the brain, behind and above the pituitary gland. Because the pineal is bathed in highly charged cerebrospinal fluid and has more blood flow per cubic volume than any other organ, it may well be the gland with the highest concentration of energy in the body.

In addition to its high concentrations of CSF and blood, the pineal gland is also the dominant source of the body's melatonin.

Melatonin and the Pineal Gland

Melatonin is significant for its effects on our mood, immune function, circadian rhythms, and the quality and quantity of our sleep. Melatonin is known as an anti-aging and anti-stress agent because it both suppresses cortisol and is a powerful antioxidant.

The production of melatonin by the pineal gland is stimulated by darkness and inhibited by light. Once released, melatonin circulates through the brain via the CSF and enters nearby blood vessels for distribution to the rest of the body. When melatonin levels are disrupted, people can experience mood swings, depression, and seasonal disorders.

Serotonin and Other Neurochemicals

In addition to producing melatonin, the pineal also metabolizes other neurochemicals that coordinate physical and emotional processes on a cellular level. These neurochemicals, including pinoline and DMT, are said to connect the mind and body. The pineal plays a key role in the production of these neurochemicals because it has one of the highest concentrations of serotonin in the body, and serotonin is a critical precursor to them.

Spiritual Aspects of the Pineal Gland

Given its important role, it is not surprising that the pineal gland has been connected with spirituality for millennia. Its pinecone shape* is found in art and artifacts of many ancient traditions, where it is associated with enlightenment and immortality (fig. 7.3). Ancient Egyptians revered this tiny gland and even preserved it separately during the process of mummification.

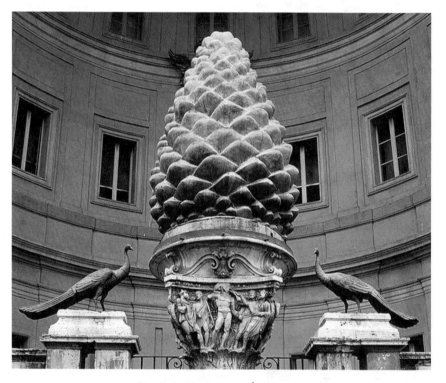

Fig. 7.3. Pinecone in the Vatican

---

*The name *pineal* is derived from the Latin word for "pinecone."

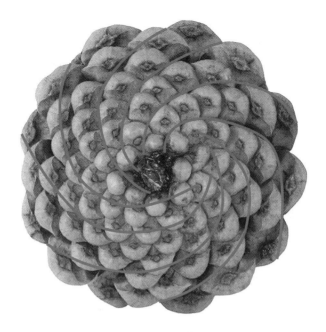

Fig. 7.4. Fibonacci spiral in a pinecone

With its spines and spirals, the pinecone illustrates a perfect Fibonacci sequence—symbolizing growth and the unifying force that underlies creation (fig. 7.4).

The Pineal Is Our Third Eye

Spiritual traditions associate the pineal with the third eye of inner vision, insight, and wisdom. Scientific research is beginning to validate the relationship between the pineal gland and vision: comparative research into the anatomy, physiology, and biochemistry of the pineal gland and the retina across a wide range of animal species suggests that the two organs share evolutionary and developmental paths. Modern living fossils such as the tuatara have a photosensitive pineal eye with a rudimentary lens, cornea, and retina. Other species such as frogs and lampreys also have pineal eyes. In humans, pineal cells resemble retinal cells in composition and in the presence of proteins not found elsewhere in the body. Pineal light sensitivity is common across diverse species.

Melatonin and the Spirit

In terms of spiritual experience, melatonin quiets the body and mind, allowing access to higher consciousness. Both pinoline and DMT are psychoactive, causing changes in perception, mood, consciousness, cognition, and behavior. Pinoline enables visions and dream states in the conscious mind and has been used by ancient Egyptians and Zoroastrians in their rituals. It assists in DNA replication and is said to resonate with the pulse of life at ~8 cycles per second.

DMT is produced during deep meditation and extraordinary conditions of birth, sexual ecstasy, extreme physical stress, and near-death experiences. It also alters our dream consciousness when it is released into the bloodstream during the Rapid Eye Movement phase of sleep. DMT links the body and spirit because of its relationship to visionary experiences and nonordinary states of transcendant consciousness. Dr. Rick Strassman calls DMT the Spirit Molecule (fig. 7.5).[1]

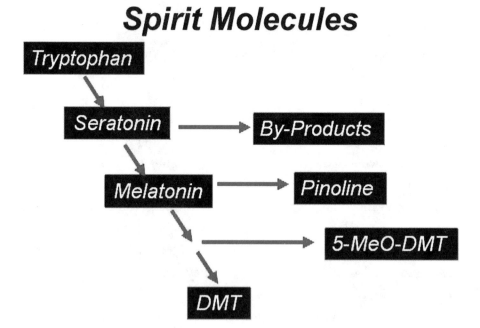

Fig. 7.5. Production path of tryptamine, serotonin, melatonin, pinoline, and DMT

The Pineal Gland and Vibration

The pineal gland can also influence our experience through vibration. As we saw earlier with the heart, rhythmic vibrations can have a powerful effect on our cognition, emotions, and physical state. We know this intuitively, and we experience it directly when we sense the effects that music has our mood, memory, and physiology. In the early 1980s, the French musician Fabien Maman researched the effect of sound vibrations on cells; he found that sounds can destroy cancer cells and invigorate healthy ones. Today, it is common for parents to play classical music to stimulate brain development in their children before and after birth.

Rhythm entrainment, also called *resonance,* happens when two wave forms begin to oscillate together at exactly the same rate. When the hypothalamus and pituitary entrain with the pulsing vibration of the pineal, our whole system can shift toward harmony.

Taoists believe that the North Star is the source of the original pulse. Vibrations from this star were crucial in the evolution of the first forms of life on Earth. It is said that Earth's ability to support life is related to the planet's tilt toward the North Star (rather than being oriented directly toward the sun). This orientation maximizes the habitable surface and optimizes the environment for plant and animal life. Because of the North Star's strong power and influence, many Chi Kung exercises intentionally connect with the North Star. According to Taoists, the North Star emits pulsing vibrations which affect the pineal gland. When the pineal pulses in synchrony with the North Star, it receives cosmic information and relays it to the hypothalamus and pituitary through resonance. In turn, they send messages to the heart which communicates with the rest of the body through its own electromagnetic pulsing.

Magnetic Fields and the Pineal Gland

Besides being sensitive to light and vibration, the pineal reacts to magnetic fields. Studies with birds and other animals conclude that the pineal gland monitors magnetic fields and assists the body in orienting in space, by acting as a navigational center. This magnetoreceptive capacity also explains why geomagnetic storms and environmental stress can affect the pineal, leading to problems with circadian rhythms and melatonin secretion.

As we discussed earlier, the heart generates a strong electromagnetic field that permeates the whole body. When the heart is activated with the high frequencies of love and compassion, its electromagnetic field is amplified and expanded. The pineal gland's sensitivity to electromagnetic energy causes it to begin vibrating in concert with the heart (fig. 7.6). As these two organs entrain together, their high vibration opens the inner eye to greater inspiration, intuition, and inner vision. Because of the pineal's connection with spatial orientation and circadian rhythms, our perception of space and time often shifts when the pineal is in a highly aroused state. Such experiences have been mentioned by meditators and Chi Kung practitioners for millennia, and research is now providing explanations for these phenomena.

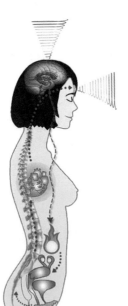

Fig. 7.6. Heart and pineal connection

THE CRYSTAL PALACE

Hypothalamus, Pituitary, and Pineal

In Taoist practices, the region of the brain bounded by the pineal, the pituitary, and hypothalamus glands is called the Crystal Palace (fig. 7.7). The Crystal Palace sits between the left and right hemispheres of the brain and between the forebrain of reason and the hind brain of instinct. Many meditation practices mention the Crystal Palace, but some people have difficulty sensing it because these structures are inside the skull and cannot be touched directly.

However, with a little practice, it is simple to connect with these glands through our awareness and intention. The location of the pineal gland is often described as the center of the head—it is at the level of the eyebrows, above and behind the pituitary and hypothalamus. Behind the eyes, the optic nerves cross at the optic chiasm. Below the optic chiasm is the pituitary gland, which sits in the sella turcica of the sphenoid. Above and behind the optic chiasm is the hypothalamus.

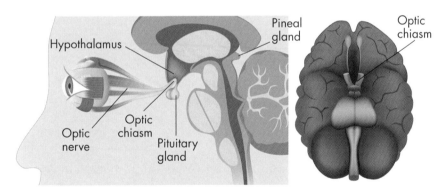

Fig. 7.7. Location of the Crystal Palace

Relationship with Light

All three glands of the Crystal Palace are extremely sensitive and responsive to light. Prior to 2002, science was aware of two forms of light receptors in the eye: cones (for color vision) and rods (for low light vision). In 2002, however, scientists discovered a third photoreceptor:

cells in the retina that contain a light-sensitive pigment called melanopsin.[2] These cells send messages to the suprachiasmatic nucleus (SCN) of the hypothalamus. The SCN is responsible for controlling circadian rhythms, which influence our sleep, alertness, hormones, temperature, and digestive functions.

When the hypothalamus receives information about the presence or absence of light, it signals the pineal to start or inhibit cortisol and melatonin production. Variation in melatonin levels causes a cascade of changes in the SCN, pituitary, and retina. The pituitary also responds to light through its release of vasopressin, which influences the SCN to adjust our circadian clock.

In addition to the light detected by our eyes, studies now show that the whole body acts as a light receptor. Light shining on any part of the body can be detected, signaling the SCN and pineal to shut down melatonin production. Because there is so much ambient light these days, our systems rarely receive the deep relaxation that occurs in total darkness. Many people find that removing light sources from the bedroom can be helpful in optimizing sleep cycles and improving general health.

Chi Kung Activates the Crystal Palace

Many chi kung practices contain simple elements like breathing or tapping that can be used to activate the bones and glands of the Crystal Palace (figs. 7.8 and 7.9).

- **Breathing:** Various breath practices move the pumps, awakening the pituitary and pineal glands as well as stimulating the flow of cerebrospinal fluid. Breathing is said to ionize the CSF and therefore increase its potency.
- **Tapping:** Gently tapping your forehead in between your eyebrows activates all three structures of the Crystal Palace. The vibration sends a wave directly back to the pineal. The same vibration also moves through the bones to the sphenoid, which in turn stimulates the pituitary gland that rests in the sella

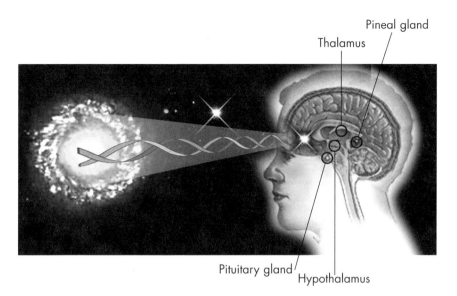

Fig. 7.8. Connecting with the Crystal Palace

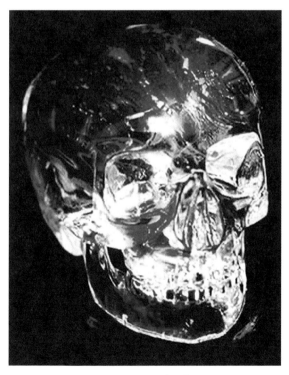

Fig. 7.9. Crystal Palace

turcica. The vibration of the pituitary awakens the hypothalamus through the pituitary stalk.

- **Toning:** Toning or chanting sends vibrations into the Crystal Palace, awakening the glands and energizing the CSF. Chanting the eight forces of the pakua to draw in elemental energies is an exceptionally powerful exercise for activating the Crystal Palace. See *Cosmic Fusion* (Destiny Books, 2007) for complete instructions on chanting the eight forces.

- **Pressing:** Pressing your tongue to the roof of your mouth activates the pituitary gland and, through its physical and chemical connections, arouses the hypothalamus and pineal glands as well.

- **Squeezing:** When we squeeze our eyes, the muscular connection with the sphenoid activates the pituitary. Sucking in our cheeks moves the jaw, which stimulates the neck and cranial pumps. Contracting the anal sphincter and perineum sends vibrations to the muscles that envelop the anus and form the pelvic floor. From the pelvis, the vibration then travels up the spine and dural tube to the occiput. The intracranial membrane system transfers the vibration to the center of the head, arousing the pineal and pituitary glands.

- **Spiraling:** Spiraling movements such as spinning the pakua, the Tai Chi symbol, or our tan tiens creates an electromagnetic field that energizes the CSF and enhances the power of the heart field.

- **Being in Darkness:** Darkness triggers increased production and release of melatonin, and eventually of pinoline and DMT.

- **Laughing and Smiling:** Smiling opens both the heart and the crown, allowing more light to penetrate while also increasing the vibration of the organs. Laughing and smiling reduce stress and relax the body, which increases the flow of chi. Laughter also triggers the release of endorphins, promoting feelings of well-being. Relaxation increases blood flow, which amplifies the effects of the hormones released in the Crystal Palace.

- **Focusing:** Since energy flows where our attention goes, bringing our attention to the structures of the Crystal Palace will activate them.

Note: The Tao also emphasizes the importance of good diet and hydration. We are 70–80 percent water, and water is highly conductive. To increase the activation of the Crystal Palace, sufficient hydration is critical. Additionally, a good, balanced diet high in tryptophan is helpful in providing the building blocks for these important biochemicals. Tryptophan is plentiful in many foods including chocolate, seaweed, almonds, bananas, dried dates, sesame seeds, chickpeas, and peanuts.

NATURAL SPIRITUAL EXPERIENCE
Chi Kung through the Eyes of Craniosacral Science

To understand how profound these Chi Kung practices are and how they kindle a natural spiritual experience, let us look at what happens with the Spinal Cord Breathing exercise introduced earlier.

As we practice Spinal Cord Breathing, the rhythmic pulsing of the spinal cord creates an electromagnetic field that charges the cerebrospinal fluid and enhances the circulation of this important fluid. Increased flow shifts the electrolyte balance, the means by which the CSF regulates the body's ability to conduct electricity. The greater the conductivity, the more energy can flow through the nervous system, charging the cells and priming them for activation. Any psychoactive substances (such as DMT) that are released by the pineal gland also enter into the CSF, charging it even further.

In Spinal Cord Breathing, the movement of the sacrum transfers vibration up the spine and to the occiput through the dural tube. Connected with the occiput at the sphenobasilar joint (SBJ), the sphenoid also begins to vibrate, stimulating the pituitary. At the same time, the rocking wavelike movement of the pituitary stalk activates the hypothalamus and milks the pituitary gland. The milking of the pituitary releases more oxytocin and vasopressin, which heighten feelings of trust, relaxation, peace, and empathy while reducing fear, anxiety, and aggression.

The pituitary gland is located above the sphenoid sinus, which drains almost directly down the throat. During high levels of excitement, CSF may be excreted into the sphenoid sinus. Here, vasopressin and oxytocin mix with the already highly charged CSF and drip down into the throat, giving us the nectar that is often described in spiritual experiences. Both vasopressin and oxytocin are critical hormones during the birth process; their presence in the nectar may contribute to birthlike experiences. The effects of these hormones on bonding may also explain the feeling of deep connection and unconditional love that is part of many enlightenment experiences.

This potent brew travels down the back of the throat and into the stomach, where it is absorbed directly through the mucous membranes. Some of this fluid also enters the bloodstream later in the digestive process. In this way, the nectar is brought to the lower tan tien for integration into the physical body, uniting heaven and earth.

During spiritual experiences, the pineal gland affects the rest of the brain through its influence on CSF, which completely immerses both the brain and the spinal cord. After bathing the brain, approximately half of the CSF gets reabsorbed into the bloodstream in the head. The other half leaves the head through lymphatic drainage. From the lymph, the supercharged CSF enters the body's bloodstream and is carried to the heart. Blood flows through the heart and vessels in a spiral motion, boosting the CSF's electromagnetic charge. These neural, biochemical, and electromagnetic connections between the brain and heart may lead to ecstatic heart-mind expanding sensations.

The heart field is the strongest electromagnetic field of the body: when consciousness moves from the head to the heart, the field becomes stronger and more organized. When the head resonates with the heart's vibration, neurons in the brain fire differently, reducing mind chatter and increasing the communication between mind and body. Thus, during spiritual experiences, the liquid-light ambrosia of the CSF is active in all three tan tiens, enhancing their powers. Because the pineal gland is itself bathed in CSF, there can be a self-amplifying positive feedback loop that creates peak experiences. Moreover, since the heart field extends and can be felt at least ten feet from the body, our experiences also have the potential for a ripple effect to our communities.

Lights and Music

Research by neurosurgeon Wilder Penfield reported in 1958 that stimulation of the right temporal lobe of the brain led to patients reporting spiritual experiences such as seeing God, leaving their bodies, hearing music, and seeing the dead.[3] Since then, studies by Peter Fenwick and Vernon Neppe also show connections between mystical experiences and the temporal lobes.[4] Although the exact mechanism by which the temporals are stimulated is not yet known, it may be that the CSF present in the interpeduncular cistern situated between the temporal lobes may be involved.

A structure called the colliculus helps to orient the head to what is seen or heard. It receives visual and auditory stimuli and has sensorimotor connections to assist with orienting movement. It surrounds the pineal gland and is affected by its secretions. As the pineal awakens, releasing biochemicals such as serotonin, tryptamine, pinoline, melatonin, or DMT, it affects the colliculus, which can explain some of the lights, visions, and celestial music that people report when the Crystal Palace is active.

JOINING THE FLOW

As we can see, Flow is critical in our lives. Although we tend to view ourselves as solid, we are actually fluid energy beings. When we perceive ourselves in this way, we become more supple, adaptable, and open to change. The more we understand about the currents running around us and through us, the more effectively we can expand our experience of them.

Understanding the Various Waves and Tides

In chapter 1, we introduced the four waves and tides used in Craniosacral Work to distinguish different types of Flow: the Cranial Wave, Fluid Tide, Long Tide, and Long Wave. In this next section, we will explore each of these in more depth, linking them to various states of consciousness.

Cranial Wave

In chapters 2 and 3, we developed our ability to perceive the Cranial Wave, the fluctuating field of energy that moves the bones and CSF. Although it can sometimes be slower, the Cranial Wave typically flows through us at about 8–14 cycles per minute or about 6 seconds per cycle. The state of our Cranial Wave indicates the health of our nervous system. Because it is an expression of our ordinary consciousness and is affected by traumas, toxins, and physical health, the Cranial Wave can be more variable than the other waves we will discuss (fig. 7.10). Therefore, we may notice frequent changes in its tempo, quality, and magnitude. At any one moment, the Cranial Wave can vary from one part of the body to another depending on the stress or health of the

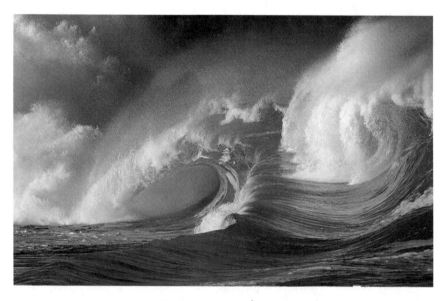

Fig. 7.10. Cranial Wave

area. When we are in Cranial Wave, we are in the active/doing phase of our practice, focusing on stimulating, balancing, and harmonizing our different parts and levels.

Fluid Tide

In contrast, the Fluid Tide is a tide-like energy field that can be sensed within the fluids and fields around the body. When we tap into the Fluid Tide, we perceive the whole unified field of the body, not just the movement of individual parts (fig. 7.11). The Fluid Tide is more stable in tempo, moving through us at 1–3 cycles per minute, roughly 24 seconds per cycle. It wells up and recedes, sweeping through us like the ocean tide. When we are in Fluid Tide, we are in a relaxed meditative state of consciousness where our power and potential are easier to access. We feel as if we are fluid. This tide tends to well up from the midline of the body on its own. The Fluid Tide reflects our deeper levels of health and healing. In chapter 6, we experienced the wholeness of the Fluid Tide within the larger flows of the Microcosmic Orbit and the meridian circulation practice.

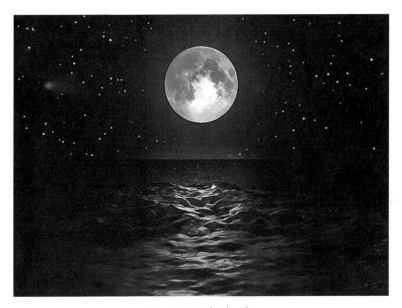

Fig. 7.11. Fluid Tide

Long Tide

The third wave observed by craniosacral practitioners is the Long Tide—an expression of the Breath of Life (fig. 7.12). The Long Tide is not affected by our history or our physical, emotional, or mental states; it moves at a stable rate of 100 seconds per cycle. This tide is often perceived as a pervasive radiance that seems to come from the horizon and move through everything. The Long Tide embodies dream or visionary consciousness, putting us in touch with deep cosmic wisdom.

In the Cranial Wave and Fluid Tide, we perceive ourselves on a personal level as individual beings. In the oceanic Long Tide, on the other hand, we experience a transpersonal consciousness in which we feel deeply interconnected with other people, our communities, the world, and the universe. We may experience this expanded state as profoundly peaceful, and we may also feel sensations of unconditional love. In Long Tide, all we need to do is open our awareness to the greater flows around us and connect with them. We become liquid light. Simply being in the Long Tide is nourishing, healing, and rejuvenating.

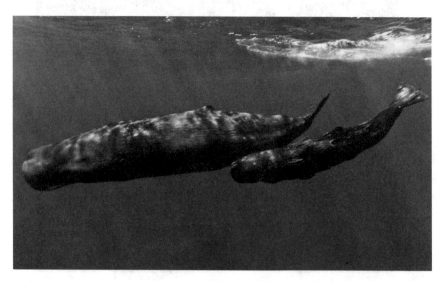

Fig. 7.12. Long Tide

Long Wave

In the Visionary CranioSacral Work taught by Hugh Milne, the fourth type of flow is the Long Wave (fig. 7.13). In Long Wave, we do not just feel connected with others, we feel One with them. In this state of unity, there is no perception of self and other, only Oneness. We are completely entrained across time and distance with a unified field of intelligent cosmic consciousness and light. We are in a state of light, Oneness, and cosmic Flow. In this Flow, we may be active; we may be still. In all cases, we Are.

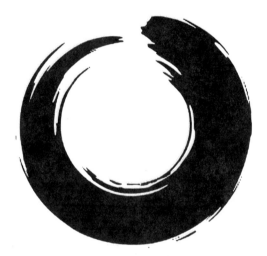

Fig. 7.13. Long Wave

Putting It All Together

If we use the metaphor of the ocean, the Cranial Wave is like the surface waves. These waves may be smooth or choppy, depending on many factors such as the wind and the landscape. Fluid Tide is like the ocean tides that ebb and flow. They move to a slower, more consistent rhythm that is connected to larger forces. The Long Tide is like the deep ocean currents that connect everything and seem to move to an ancient timeless rhythm. The Long Wave may feel so all-encompassing that it may feel like an enfoldment more than a movement.

A Balanced Approach to Joining the Flow

The transition from ordinary consciousness concerned with work, relationships, and daily life to cosmic consciousness or even transpersonal consciousness can be challenging. Although we may want to dive into the experience, in order to minimize frustration it is best not to rush. Appreciate and enjoy the benefits of the warm-up practices that balance our different layers and levels. They are not only valuable in and of themselves, but they also provide useful preparation for what follows.

Without harmonizing our physical, emotional, and mental layers, it can be difficult to access our energy and spiritual aspects because the areas that are out of balance demand too much attention and chi. It is also important to have a strong and stable foundation so that the extraordinary experiences of these nonordinary states do not create imbalances; we need to be able to integrate our experiences smoothly.

The Tao teaches us the principle of balanced yin and yang: to go up, we must go down; to go forward, we must go back; to go out, we must go in. In terms of application, this means that if we want to expand our consciousness up and out to the cosmos, we need to be very well grounded and rooted within ourselves (fig. 7.14). Many of us want

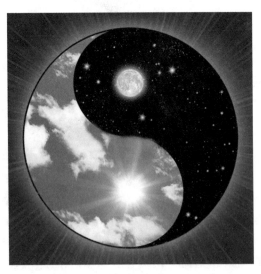

Fig. 7.14. A balanced approach

to go on cosmic journeys because we are unhappy here on Earth in our earthly bodies. In such circumstances, our quest for spirituality may come from unhappiness with this world rather than from excitement and interest in something more. We look outside because we do not want to look inside. If this is the case, then we may tend to leave our bodies when we travel the cosmos. However, it is important to understand that the physical body is our temple and also our source of energy. If we become disconnected from it and do not take good care of ourselves, then before long, we will not have enough energy for the journey.

Therefore, rather than leaving or ignoring our bodies, the optimal approach is to take time to integrate our inner selves as part of our quest to connect with the cosmos. It is better to remain a resident of the earth plane and expand our consciousness upward and outward from this stable foundation.

Looking again at the ancient Taoist painting of the water wheel, we can see the mountains at the top reaching to the North Star (fig. 7.15).

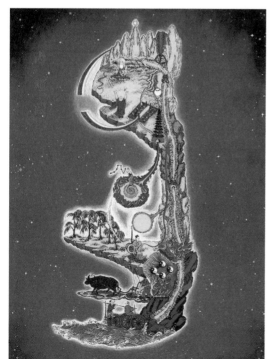

Fig. 7.15. Cosmic wisdom

Like the figures in the painting, we can remain on earth, extending our antenna up into the heavens to connect with the cosmic internet and download universal wisdom into our consciousness. Although it is also possible to build a rocket ship and explore the universe, the approach of staying connected to earth and our body while expanding out into the cosmos is easier, safer, and takes a lot less effort.

THE WORLD LINK
MEDITATION

In this section, we will use the World Link meditation as an opportunity to experience being liquid light. We will begin the meditation by activating, balancing, and harmonizing our energy. Then we'll move the energy through our whole system to increase Flow before expanding our awareness to our communities and the cosmos.

It is important to note that while we sometimes may notice things as they are happening, the true effects of a practice are often more noticeable after we've stopped *doing* and are simply resting and being. This is especially true in the beginning when we are just learning a new practice: we may be so focused on doing things correctly that we feel more of the effects as we rest afterward.

Warm-Ups for the World Link Meditation

Sensing the Cranial Wave

1. Stand comfortably with your feet shoulder-width apart and your knees slightly bent. Bring your head into alignment with your heart and your sacrum.
2. Begin natural breathing. Feel the inhalation (yang) and the exhalation (yin). Let your breathing become slower, smoother, and more even, bringing balance to yin and yang and to the Flow

that connects and transforms them from one to the other.

3. Do 9 rounds of slow, gentle Spinal Cord Breathing to awaken your pumps and increase the flow of cerebrospinal fluid. Feel the CSF flowing between your sacrum and your head.

Combining the Three Tan Tiens

Moving into Fluid Tide

1. Relax the abdomen and smile golden sunshine down to the lower tan tien. Activate the tan tien energy until your navel feels full and warm. Observe the power and rootedness of your lower tan tien. Bring your awareness to the Door of Life/Ming Men behind your navel; activate your Kidney Chi. Notice the vitality you feel when your lower burner is activated and the energy is flowing through Ming Men and your tan tien.

2. Now bring your awareness to your heart and activate its power. Feel the heart full of love, joy, and happiness. Notice how smiling and feeling love amplifies the heart field. As the flow in your heart center increases, feel your emotions harmonizing.

3. Smile into your head and breathe deeply in and out. Let the slow rhythm of your breath ease any tension in the head. Feel your thoughts quieting and flowing more peacefully.

4. Empty your head by inviting the smiling energy to spiral down from it to your chest and into your heart. Feel the spiraling motion charge the CSF.

5. Spiral the head and Heart Chi into the tan tien (see fig. 7.16 on page 216). Fuse the three brains together into one mind/Yi. Bring the power of the Yi to the third eye point. Feel your third eye and pineal activating. Rest for several moments here, enjoying the feeling of balanced harmonious Flow throughout your entire being. Feel your health and wholeness.

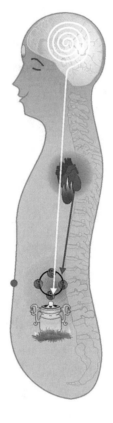

Fig. 7.16. Universal World
Link and the Fluid Tide

 Expanding to the Six Directions

Connecting to the Long Tide

Now we will expand our unified mind/Yi to connect with the cosmic
forces and the Long Tide.

1. **Front/Back:** Open your awareness to the universe in front of you
   and the universe behind you. Inhale. As you exhale, extend your
   hands to the front by pushing your palms outward (fig. 7.17a).
   Expand and connect with the cosmos and infinite space. Imagine
   there are small vacuum points in the center of your palms. As you
   exhale, let your elbows sink and the vacuums in your palms draw
   energy into your hands, through your arms, and down to your tan
   tien (fig. 7.17b). Feel the cosmic light entering into your energy
   field, increasing your vibration.

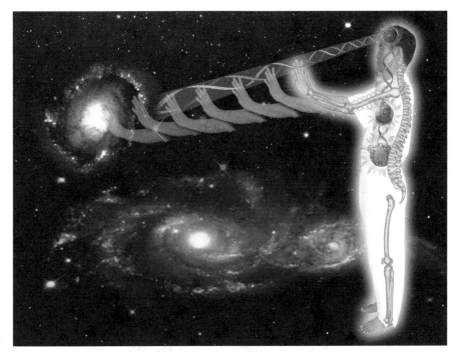

A

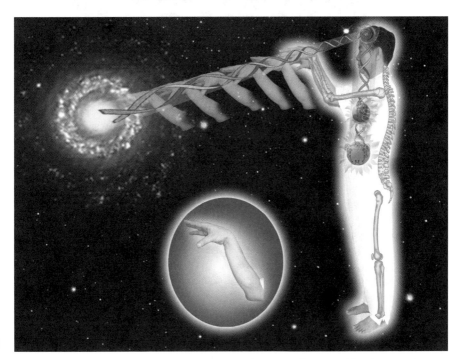

B

Fig. 7.17. Connecting with universal energy, front and back

2. **Left/Right:** Open your awareness and connect with the universe on each side. Bend your elbows and bring your hands to the sides of your shoulders with your palms facing outward. Inhale. As you exhale, extend your palms out to the sides (fig. 7.18a). Connect with the horizon and the cosmos beyond. On inhalation, let your elbows bend and your hands move back toward your shoulders (fig. 7.18b). Draw in cosmic energy through the vacuum points in the center of your palms, into your hands and arms, and then down into your tan tien. Feel the amplification of your internal light.

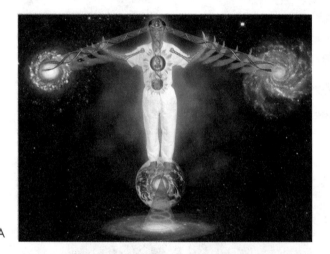

A

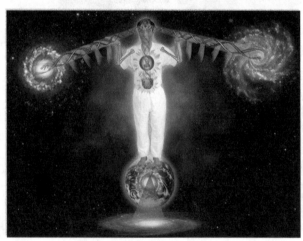

B

Fig. 7.18. Connecting with universal energy, right and left

3. **Above/Below:** Expand your awareness to the universe above and below. Turn your palms up. As you inhale, raise your palms up to the cosmos (fig. 7.19). Scoop up the chi. As you exhale, draw the chi in through your crown all the way down to your perineum, then down through the earth to the universe below. Let the Cosmic Chi awaken your Crystal Palace. Feel your pineal, pituitary, and hypothalamus glands pulsing in synchrony. Notice your heart expanding. Feel your heart entraining with the Crystal Palace and sense them pulsing together.

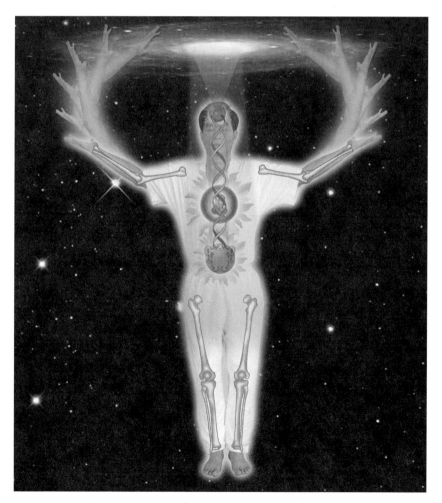

Fig. 7.19. Connecting with universal energy, above and below

4. **Eat the Cosmos:** Move your tongue around your mouth 9 times in one direction, then 9 times in the opposite direction. Tap your teeth together 9 times. Then swallow your saliva and any nectar from the Crystal Palace down into your lower tan tien.

5. **Integrate:** Rest for a moment, feeling yourself bathed in cosmic energy and light from the six directions. Feel your CSF increasing its potency, pulsing with its own radiance in tune with the heart and Crystal Palace.

6. **Connect with your personal star:** With the power of your Yi/ united mind, open your awareness to your personal star 6 inches above your head. Your personal star is a focal point from which you can expand your consciousness out to the whole universe.

7. **Connect with your community:** Expand your awareness to your community. Spiral out and link with everyone's personal star (fig. 7.20).

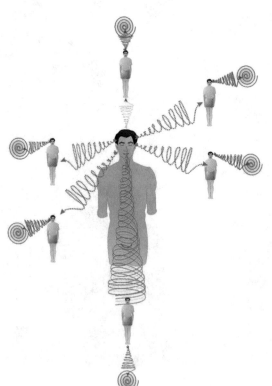

Fig. 7.20. Connect with your community.

8. **Connect with the universe:** Feel rays of light connecting you with others. Then feel the matrix of personal stars spiraling up to connect with the heart of the universe (fig. 7.21). Feel yourself as part of the matrix of the universe, of All That Is. Notice the sense of dynamic movement and Flow and melt into it until you become liquid light.

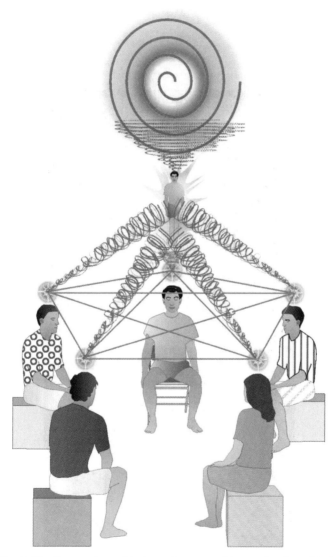

Fig. 7.21. Connecting with the universe and becoming liquid light

9. **Breathe, listen, sense, feel:** Visualization becomes actualization. At some point, you no longer need to visualize being connected to others and the universe because you *are* connected to the universe. Simply breathe. There is nothing we really need to do other than to open our awareness and tune in. Once we have done that, our work is over.

At some point, you may notice that you are not breathing; the cosmic force is breathing you. This is the Breath of Life. It flows around us and through us. And if we allow it, this cosmic Flow moves us toward health, harmony, and wholeness with its cosmic wisdom (fig. 7.22).

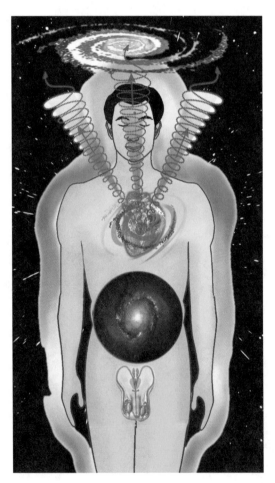

Fig. 7.22. Cosmic connection

Chuang Tzu taught us that those who practice the Tao do less and less every day until they reach a point where they do nothing (fig. 7.23). Nothing is done, yet nothing is left undone.

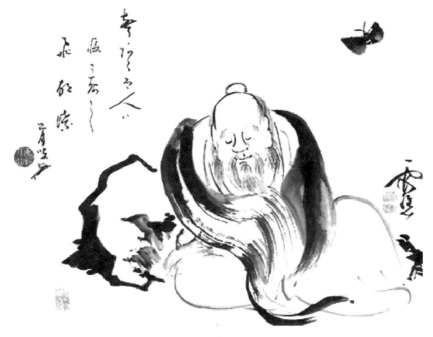

Fig. 7.23. Chuang Tzu

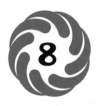

Cosmic Flow

The Art and Skill of Nondoing

In this fast-paced, busy world, nondoing can be a difficult, yet worth-while practice. We are taught that to be successful we need to work hard and do more. While it is true that there are times when action is necessary, there are also times when the fruits of our action ripen in the space and stillness of nonaction. In Taoism, this principle of action and nonaction is known as *Wu Wei*.

Wu Wei is the principle of yang and yin: doing and not doing. In the moment of maximum yang, there is always the seed of yin and vice versa. Stillness and quiet naturally follow from activity and, even in what seems like stillness, activity is arising. The alchemical transformation back and forth between yin and yang occurs naturally all the time and is necessary for balance and true health. Rather than forcing, rushing, or restraining this natural Flow, we can optimize ourselves by understanding this foundational principle and allowing it to guide us back to harmony.

For many people, knowing when to do and when not to do can be challenging. Both Taoism and Craniosacral Work teach us that change and deep healing often occur when we surrender to the Flow and let go of making an effort. Transitioning smoothly and effectively between yang and yin is more skill and art than a rote process.

Yin and Yang Breathing

We can develop our consciousness and skills with the simple abdominal breathing practice we introduced earlier (fig. 8.1).

1. Sit or stand comfortably with your spine aligned.
2. Invite your tailbone to connect with the earth and your crown to connect with the North Star.

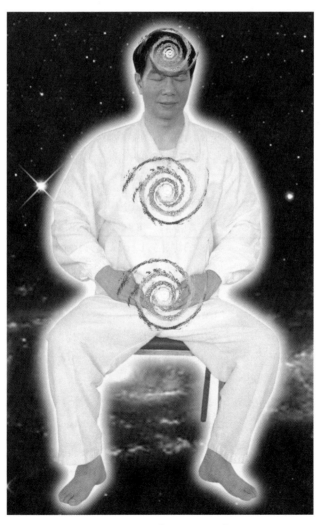

Fig. 8.1. Yin and Yang Breathing

3. Begin abdominal breathing. As you inhale, let your abdomen expand. As you exhale, let it move back toward your spine.

4. Invite your breath to slow and become more smooth and even. Take 9 breaths, each one slower and longer than the one before. This is the Cranial Wave.

5. Bring your awareness to your inhalations. Notice the sensations as you approach your maximum inhalation and pause slightly before allowing the exhalation to begin.

6. Exhale fully and without effort or rushing. Notice the sensations as you approach your maximum exhalation and pause for a moment before initiating the inhalation.

7. Observe the space in between inhalation and exhalation. Let go of making the pause happen and just feel the transition between yang and yin. You may feel as if you are floating during the change. It is a place where yang flows seamlessly into yin and yin into yang, expansion into contraction into expansion in an ongoing effortless cycle. This is the Fluid Tide.

8. As you rest in your breath, your mind becomes more quiet and tranquil. Your emotions become more balanced and peaceful. Your body relaxes and releases. All this happens without effort.

9. As you continue breathing, you may reach a point where you feel like you are being breathed rather than doing the breathing. Your whole system is breathing, expanding, and contracting with the Breath of Life. The Primordial Force is doing the breathing for you. Relax. Allow. Become the Flow. This is the Long Tide.

10. Smile. Allow your awareness to expand. Become aware of your heart tilted to the North Star and feel its pulse. The pulses of the North Star, Vega, and Thuban affect the earth's pulse (fig. 8.2). Feel the pulse; allow and invite the Flow to increase.

11. Bring your attention to your skin, which is the physical boundary between you and not-you. You may notice that your breath slows so much that it seems to stop. Your lungs are no longer breathing; your skin is breathing. The boundary between you and not-you

dissolves. You expand and become One with the universe. Perhaps there is a sensation of motion or perhaps there is stillness. It is a dynamic stillness of infinite potential. Craniosacral workers call this Long Wave; Taoists call it Wu Ji.

12. Rest in this state of Being until you are complete.

13. Return to abdominal breathing. Gather your energy and store it in your lower tan tien.

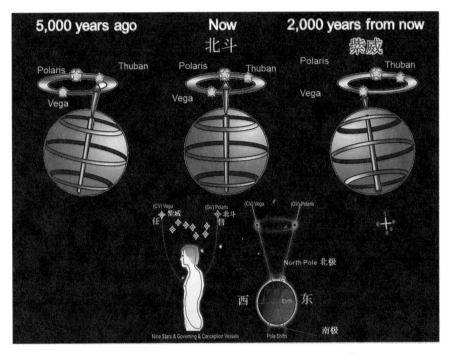

Fig. 8.2. The pulses of the North Star, Vega, and
Thuban affect the earth's pulse.

In the previous exercise, we increased our capacity to sense the transitions between yin and yang. We practiced relaxing into fluidity and joining the larger flows until we became the Flow. Being able to join the Flow in meditation is good; being able to sense Flow in daily life is even better. To continue building our skills, we will use the following simple Chi Kung exercise.

Flowing between Empty and Full

1. Stand with your feet shoulder-width apart. Let your arms relax by your sides.
2. Connect the soles of your feet with the earth and your crown to the North Star.
3. Shift your weight slowly to your right leg, then to your left leg. Do 3 cycles. Feel the movement of the weight shifting from one leg to the other (fig. 8.3).
4. Now, as you shift your weight to the right, feel the energy travelling all the way down your leg to your foot, until 100 percent of your weight is in the right foot.
5. Begin to shift your weight to your left foot, feeling the energy rising from the bottom of your right foot up the right leg, flowing through the tan tien until it pours down the left leg to the left foot. Do 3 cycles. Notice the transition from complete yang (full weight) to complete yin (no weight) with each foot. When your weight is 100 percent on either leg, you should be able to lift the other one easily, without moving your torso.

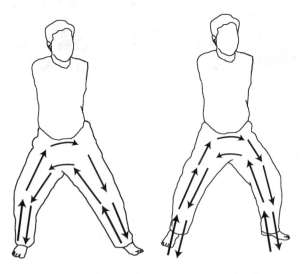

Fig. 8.3. Flowing between Empty and Full

6. The next time, slow the shifting of your weight. Allow weight to pour like honey down to your right leg until it reaches your right foot, then let it continue down deep into the earth. When it reaches its maximum depth, feel it rebounding back up the right leg. Sense it rising until it reaches your tan tien and then flows down the left leg to the left foot and into the earth. Continue for 3 full cycles. Observe as the energy reaches its maximum extension and begins to return. Notice as it moves across your pelvis and then begins to travel down the other leg. When your weight is 100 percent on one foot and the energy flows deep into the earth, the "empty" foot will feel as if it is almost lifting by itself to balance the "full" one.

7. Think of your hip as Point A and your foot as Point Z. Think of the bottom of your foot where it touches the earth as Point 0 and the maximum depth you reach in the earth as Point 100.

8. Allow the transfer of your weight and the movement of energy to slow down until you can sense the energy not only at Point A and then at Point Z, but at as many points in between as possible. Then bring more awareness to your energy as it travels between Point 0 and Point 100. This is an ongoing process of refinement. When you can sense points 1, 2, 3, and so on, then you can begin to notice points 1.25, 1.50, 1.75, etc. Notice if there are regions where your awareness disappears, and if that is consistent from day to day. Invite the light of your awareness to be steady, strong, and stable as it flows up and down your legs and your weight transfers from leg to leg. Explore increasing your awareness of the Flow in this way for another 3 cycles.

9. Now expand your awareness from the details to the bigger perspective, and let the energy move freely through your body. Notice the energy as your weight changes from side to side and follow it wherever it goes. Let go of consciously shifting your weight and move with the energy as it changes. Let go of any tension so that the flow of energy increases and you can follow it more easily.

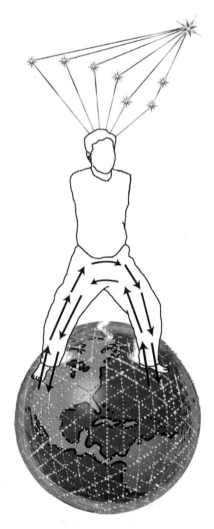

Fig. 8.4. Connecting with energy above and below

10. Connect with the earth energy below and the North Star above, then relax and let the energy move you (fig. 8.4). Just as in the natural world, there will be moments when movement subsides. When that occurs, pause until you feel the movement start again on its own.

11. Stay connected with your experience. When it feels complete, gather the energy into your lower tan tien and seal it in with 9 spirals in each direction.

Flowing between Empty to Full helps us experience the movement from yin to yang and back to yin more clearly. Every time we take a step in daily life, we are expressing and living this principle, but we may not have been aware of it before. With each step we can connect to the larger flows, and we can also observe how it feels to allow ourselves to be moved by the Tao.

Push Hands: Moving Into Stillness

In this exercise, we return to the partner Push Hands exercises we did in chapter 5 to experience the arising of stillness. This exercise gives us the opportunity to work with a partner and see how it feels to join the Flow together with another person.

1. Stand facing your partner with both hands touching your partner's hands in a palm-to-palm connection (fig. 8.5).

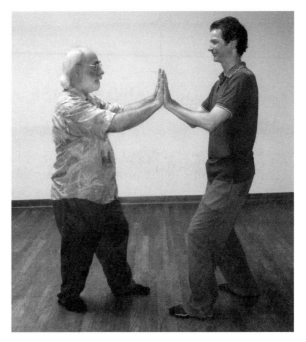

Fig. 8.5. Push Hands: Moving into Stillness

2. Relax and breathe.

3. The intention for each person is simply to listen. Listen with your hands, heart, and whole being for the Flow that you are creating together.

4. Allow movement to unfold with neither person consciously leading. Let your mind rest and release control. Simply listen and follow the Flow together. Notice what is different for you about sensing the Flow together.

5. Just as water ebbs and flows in nature, naturally arising healthy movement will vary rather than repeat continuously. Notice when the movement comes to stillness and then when it restarts again on its own. Allow yourself to rest in the stillness and to enter into movement again when it emerges.

6. Notice the dynamic quality of stillness and how the energy flow changes once the movement begins again. Allow yourselves the opportunity to be in stillness and motion for several cycles.

7. Listen for a deep stillness that marks a good place to complete this practice. Release contact with your partner.

8. Bring the energy down to your lower tan tien and rest in stillness.

PREPARE, AIM, AND RELEASE

Relaxing and joining the Flow sounds easy, but our desires and fears can make it hard for us to actually experience it. When we want something very strongly, but do not trust in the process or the outcome, then our need for control arises and we may try to manipulate the Flow. Usually this results in more tension, more effort, and less overall Flow. We can't safely force experiences to happen, especially spiritual ones. Through the Chi Kung exercises, we can become familiar with how both movement and stillness naturally arise, and that it is often in the moments after we finish "doing" the practice that Flow is greatest and we are able to access the fullest potential of what the practice has to offer. In those moments, we stop doing, stop trying, relax, and move into No Mind.

Different from mindlessness, spaciness, or apathy, No Mind is a state of openness and presence without agenda. Lao Tzu tells us that the whole universe surrenders to the mind that is still. It is in the spaciousness of No Mind that we receive the greatest benefits and truly Flow with the Tao. When we do that, we access all of our power and potential and all of the power and potential of the Universe.

The Chi Kung exercise Pull the Bow and Shoot the Arrow is one of the best practices for teaching us about doing our work, then standing back and letting go. It is a profound teaching on the process of focusing our attention, setting our intention, and relaxing into No Mind. We can also call these steps Prepare, Aim, and Release.

- **Prepare.** For our spiritual growth, we need to prepare ourselves by focusing our attention. We start by deciding what our priorities are and where we are going to put our energy. At the same time, we take care of our physical, emotional, and mental health by attending to our diet, exercise, and physical alignment. We use our Chi Kung practices and meditation to harmonize our emotional and mental aspects. And we build, cultivate, and refine our energy. This process creates more Flow throughout all of our systems.

- **Aim.** It is also important to clarify our intentions and understand why we are doing what we are doing. This is akin to identifying a target and taking aim. As we do the inner work of contemplating our motivation, assumptions, and belief systems, we get valuable insights into deeper layers of our being. Although we may or may not know the exact details, we gain a sense for how we want to grow, who we want to become, and where we are heading in our personal and spiritual development. Are we doing the practices with the intention of greater physical health, smoother relationships, peace, psychic gifts, bliss, connection with the universe, or to experience Oneness?

  Our intentions are critical because they shape our experiences and have a strong influence on the gifts and benefits that we actually receive from our practices. There are many flows in the universe, but not all of them are appropriate. Once we know our intentions, we can discern which flows we are aligned with and can enhance our own Flow.

- **Release.** By letting go it all gets done. The world is won by those who know when and how to let go. Because our attention and intentions are so powerful and so influenced by our filters, they can be both helpful and limiting. Our conscious mind is not always able to hold a broad enough perspective for us to understand Wholeness. As long as we have an agenda—any agenda—then we have a preference for an outcome. Naturally, we try to assist, control, or direct the process to achieve that outcome, and our awareness is fixed on how we are doing relative to that goal. This does not allow us to truly join the cosmic Flow.

  Once we have learned to focus our attention and have clarified our intentions we get to relax and simply Be. We prepare, aim, and then we release. The first two steps are important for achieving and manifesting in the everyday world. The final step is crucial for our longevity and spiritual growth.

Pull the Bow and Shoot the Arrow

1. Stand or sit comfortably. Fold the pinky, ring, and middle fingers of both hands to the palm. Hold your hands a few inches away from your chest in front of your sternum. Round your shoulders slightly and rotate your right hand so that the thumb turns outward and the index finger points to the left (fig. 8.6).

2. Turn your left hand so that the palm is facing the left and the index finger points upward.

3. Imagine that you are drawing a bow and fitting an arrow to your bowstring.

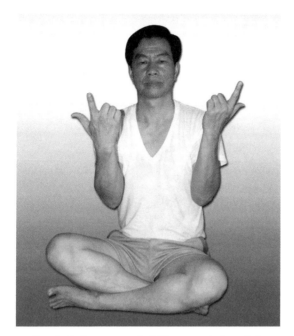

Fig. 8.6. Prepare to hold bow and shoot left.

4. Inhale. Pull your right hand back toward your ear and stretch your left hand toward your left side (fig. 8.7). Train your body. Develop your strength. Expand your energy field and get the chi flowing.

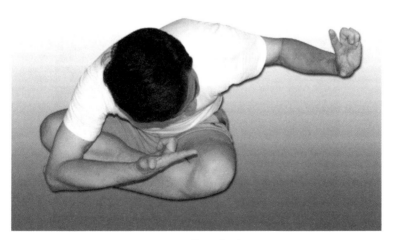

Fig. 8.7. Pulling the bow

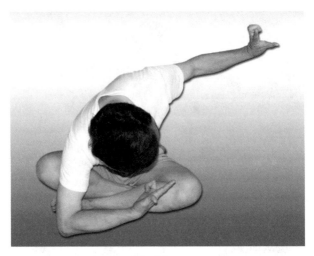

Fig. 8.8. Taking aim

5. Turn your neck and head to take aim at the target. Set your intention. Clarify your goals and know your direction (fig. 8.8).

6. Relax and release the arrow (fig. 8.9). Exhale and let go. Repeat 3, 6, or 9 times on each side, then return to center. Allow your energy to expand and flow. Relax into the space and be in your experience.

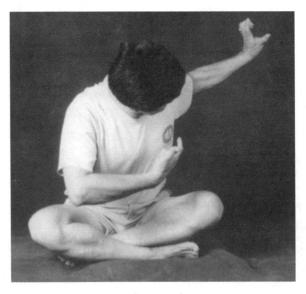

Fig. 8.9. Shooting the arrow

BECOMING THE COSMIC FLOW

When we are sick or in pain, our awareness fragments and narrows. We then tend to focus on the disharmony or problem and lose our connection to health. When we focus on nonhealth, our energy follows our attention. We expend energy getting drawn into fixing, doing, and "efforting."

When we remember to shift our consciousness to view the bigger picture, we can put the issue into perspective and sense the inherent health of the universe around us and within us. This reminder of the pervasive presence of well-being is one of the great benefits of Chi Kung practices. As we rest our awareness on health, aspects of health are amplified, facilitating a return to wholeness. Chi Kung uplifts us and reminds us that we are empowered to make choices that move us back toward that health and back into the Flow. When we become One with the cosmic Flow, we are truly healthy and whole.

Becoming the Cosmic Flow

1. Sit or stand, with your head, heart, and sacrum aligned.
2. Breathe, rock your sacrum, and squeeze your eyes and perineum to activate your pumps and enhance the flow of cerebrospinal fluid. Awaken the Flow in your physical body.
3. Bring your awareness to the swimming dragon and fire dragon to activate your spine and Crystal Palace.
4. Smile and let the smiling energy flow down into your heart.
5. Feel love, joy, and happiness in your heart. Feel your emotional and mental flows balancing and harmonizing.
6. Invite the smile down into your abdomen and continue smiling until your belly feels warm and full.
7. Let the smile transform the energy of the brain in each tan tien. Fuse the head, heart, and gut brains into one mind, Yi, at the third eye. Feel the pineal, pituitary, and hypothalamus awakening and the Crystal Palace filling with light. Feel the circulation

of energy through your meridians and Microcosmic Orbit.

8. Bring your awareness to your Personal Star, which symbolizes your intention.

9. Expand your awareness to the cosmos. Smile. Feel your smile opening your crown and connecting you to the cosmos (fig. 8.10).

10. Feel the North Star and sense it pulsing with the wisdom of the universe.

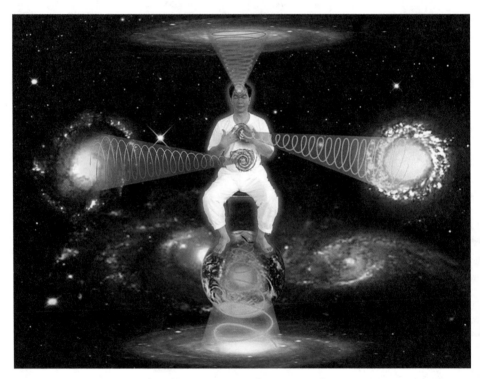

Fig. 8.10. Becoming the Cosmic Flow

11. Observe your Crystal Palace beginning to pulse in tune with the universal wisdom. Download cosmic energy and information into your crown.

12. Feel your cerebrospinal fluid pulsing together with the Crystal Palace and the North Star, absorbing and distributing liquid light throughout the whole body.

13. Notice your heart picking up the pulse and sending a resonant fre-

quency through its powerful electromagnetic field to the rest of the body. Feel all the flows joining together into one large cosmic Flow.

14. Relax and empty the mind. Let your empty mind expand to encompass the universe.

15. Feel your entire being pulsing with the pulsing of the universe until you become the Flow.

16. Flow out and in and out and in. Be present.

17. The Flow may be active at times and still at others. Relax into the Flow more deeply and let it carry you to new places.

18. Eventually, the Flow will deposit you back on the shore, in your body. When you return, rest for some moments. Notice what has shifted. Smile.

19. Collect all your energy in your tan tien and close the practice by spiraling 9 times in one direction and 9 times in the other.

The goal of Craniosacral Chi Kung is to empower people to connect with the internal flows and the greater cosmic flows that lead us back to health. To provide guidance on this journey, we have offered an abundance of practical exercises for increasing and harmonizing Flow on all levels. The practices in this book have been selected to awaken Flow and deepen practitioners' capacity to sense, track, and optimize all flows. By making the connection between ancient Chi Kung practices and the approach of Craniosacral Work, which is based on modern physiology, practitioners can better understand what these exercises were designed to do and why they work. Through practicing with increased attention and more focused intention, both beginning and advanced practitioners can reap greater benefits.

However, optimizing our growth and potential, enjoying health and happiness, and experiencing connection and Oneness do not require making a concerted effort or doing all the practices all the time! Connecting to the Tao is much easier than that. To receive those benefits, we encourage everyone to remember that all we need do is simply prepare ourselves, set our intentions, smile, and relax into the Flow.

Appendix 1

Cosmic Cranial-Elemental Connections

The Universal Healing Tao practices recognize that the cranial bones also have connections to cosmic and elemental forces (fig. A.1).

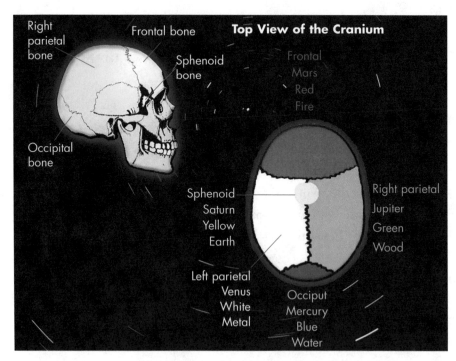

Fig. A.1. Cranial bone relationships to cosmic and elemental forces

COSMIC CRANIAL-ELEMENTAL CONNECTIONS

COSMIC CONNECTIONS	PLANET	CRANIAL BONE	ELEMENT	ORGANS, REGIONS
Northern star palace, blue galaxy	Mercury	Occiput	Water	Kidney/Bladder, bones, hormones
Eastern star palace, green galaxy	Jupiter	Right parietal	Wood	Liver/Gall Bladder, ligaments, tendons
Southern star palace, red galaxy	Mars	Frontal	Fire	Heart/Small Intestine, circulatory system
Western star palace, white galaxy	Venus	Left parietal	Metal	Lung/Large Intestine, skin
Central star palace, yellow galaxy	Saturn	Sphenoid	Earth	Spleen/Pancreas/ Stomach, muscles

 ## Cosmic Cranial-Elemental Meditation

This practice will increase the flow and harmony of the cranial-elemental connections.

1. First, activate the cranial pump by pressing the tip of your tongue to your lower jaw and the body of the tongue to your upper palate (fig. A.2).

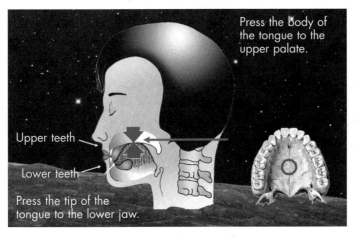

Fig. A.2. Activate the cranial pump.

2. Clench your teeth to activate the sphenoid. Drop your chin and press it backward to activate the occiput (fig. A.3).

3. Tune in to the Cranial Wave by placing your hands on your head, palms just above your ears. You can also try feeling the wave with one hand on your forehead (the frontal bone) and the other at the base of your skull (the occiput). Feel the cranial rhythm (fig. A.4).

4. Place one hand on your occiput and the other on your back over one of your kidneys. Fill your occiput and kidneys with blue light, and with the calm and gentleness of the water element. Picture Mercury as a blue ball above your occiput. Connect Mercury, the occiput, and the kidneys (fig. A.5).

5. Place one hand on your right parietal bone and the other on your liver. Fill your right parietal bone and your liver with green light, and with the friendliness of the wood element. Picture Jupiter as a

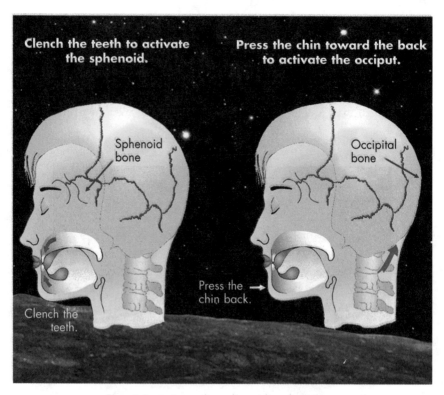

Fig. A.3. Activate the sphenoid and occiput.

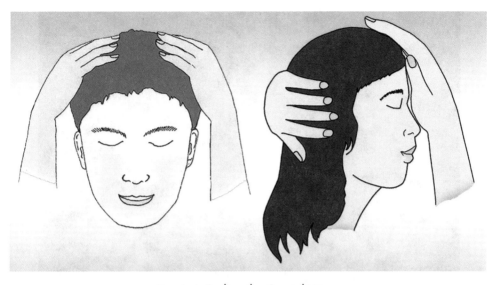

Fig. A.4. Feeling the Cranial Wave

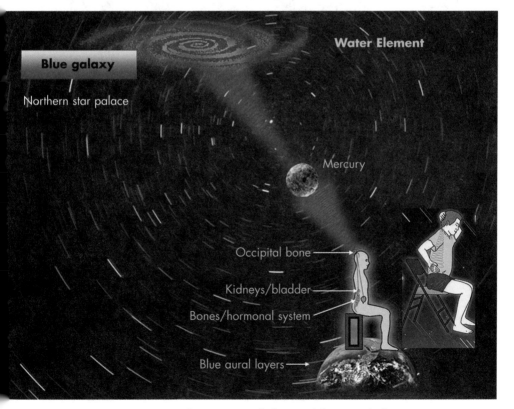

Fig. A.5. Connecting the cosmic and elemental forces with the occiput

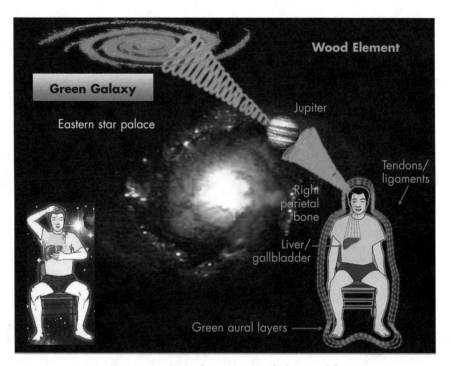

Fig. A.6. Connecting the cosmic and elemental forces
with the right parietal bone

green ball above the right parietal. Connect Jupiter, the right parietal, and the liver (fig. A.6).

6. Hold your frontal bone with one hand and your heart with the other. Fill your frontal bone and your heart with red light, and with the love, joy, and happiness of the fire element. Picture Mars as a red ball above the frontal bone. Connect Mars, the frontal bone, and your heart (fig. A.7).

7. Hold the left parietal bone and your lungs. Fill your left parietal bone and your lungs with white light, and with the courage of the metal element. Picture Venus as a white ball above your left parietal bone. Connect Venus, the left parietal, and your lungs (fig. A.8).

8. The sphenoid is in the center of the head. For this meditation, use a flat hand to hold the spleen and a beaked hand to touch the top of the head, while letting your focused intention drop into the center

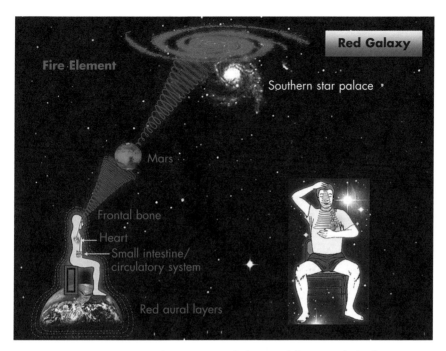

Fig. A.7. Connecting the cosmic and elemental forces with the heart

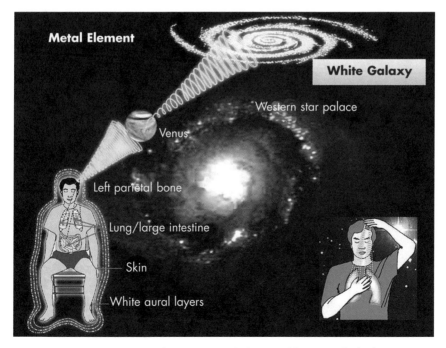

Fig. A.8. Connecting the cosmic and elemental forces with the lungs

of the head to connect with the sphenoid. Fill your spleen and sphenoid bone with yellow light, and with the fairness, openness, and trust of the earth element. Picture Saturn as a yellow ball above the top of your head and sphenoid. Connect Saturn, the sphenoid, and your spleen (fig. A.9).

9. Feel the five cosmic planetary forces connecting with the five cranial bones, the five elements, and the five organs. Feel the energies flowing in and filling bones and organs with light and chi (fig. A.10).

10. Sense the planetary forces beaming their energies and vibrations into the Crystal Palace in the center of your head.

11. Rest in the stillness and relax into the experience.

12. To close, bring the energy down from the Crystal Palace to your heart, and finally down to your lower tan tien (fig. A.11). Spiral the energy 9 times in one direction and 9 times in the other to seal the energy.

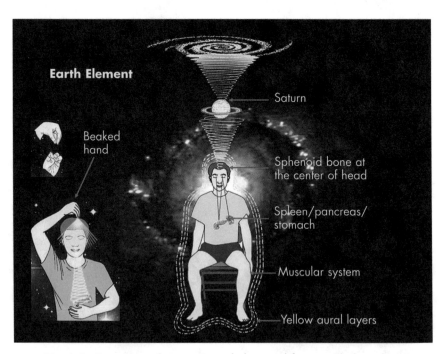

Fig. A.9. Connecting the cosmic and elemental forces with the spleen

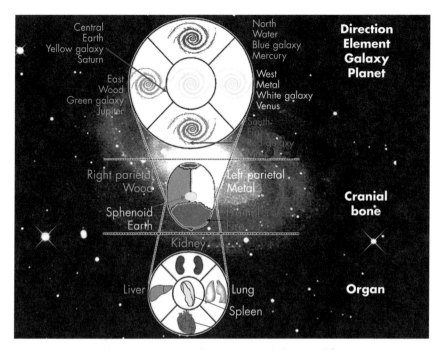

Fig. A.10. Integrating the cosmic and elemental forces

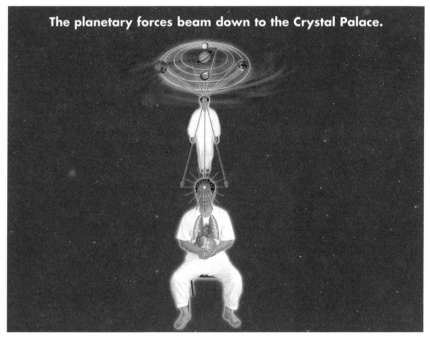

Fig. A.11. Filling the Crystal Palace, the heart, and the tan tien

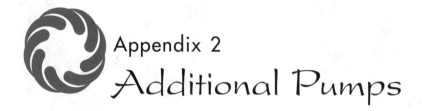

Appendix 2
Additional Pumps

This book has focused on four major pumps: the cardiac, respiratory, cranial, and sacral pumps. However, there are many more pumps in the body, and each is responsible for moving fluids and chi through our system. Good circulation means good flow, so it is important for us to keep all of our pumps active and in good working order.

A short list of the other pumps includes, but is not limited to, the following:

- Crown pump
- Temporal pump
- Cervical pump (C7)
- Middle thoracic/sternum/thymus pump
- Lower thoracic/adrenal pump (T11)
- Lumbar/Door of Life pump (L2/L3)
- Perineal, anal, scrotal, and ovarian pumps
- Abdominal pumps (stomach, liver, spleen, and pancreas)
- Lymphatic pumps in our arms and legs

Many of the Chi Kung exercises and techniques introduced in this book will also work well for activating these other important pumps. Any time we flex and compress ourselves, we squeeze blood out of an area. When we extend and expand, new blood and oxygen floods this area, energizing the pumps. Some of the key exercises are:

- Natural and Reverse Breathing for the abdominal and lymphatic pumps
- Spinal Cord Breathing/Crane/Turtle/Wagging the Tail for the lumbar, lower thoracic, middle thoracic, and cervical pumps
- Opening the Waist, Hips, and Sacrum for the perineum, lumbar, lower thoracic, and abdominal pumps
- Activating the Crystal Palace (see pages 202–4) for the perineum, abdominal, temporal, and crown pumps

Additional exercises from other books that are useful for awakening the pumps include:

- Clicking the teeth, pressing the palate, pushing the chin backward (See appendix 1) for the crown, temporal pump, and cervical pumps
- Tapping the kidneys for the adrenal pump
- Squeezing the arms, legs, and eyes for the lymph pumps
- Iron Shirt Chi Kung and Stem Cell or Bone Marrow Chi Kung for all the pumps
- Power Lock (see *Chi Kung for Prostate Health and Sexual Vigor* or *Chi Kung for Women's Health and Sexual Vitality* for detailed instructions for men and women) for the perineal, anal, scrotal, sacral, adrenal, cranial, and lymphatic pumps

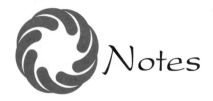

Notes

Sources preceded by an asterisk can be found in the list of online resources immediately following the bibliography.

Chapter 1. Working with Cosmic Flow

1. *LearnersDictionary.com, "Learner's definition of FLOW"; *Merriam-Webster.com, "Full Definition of Flow."

Chapter 2. Awakening the Major Pumps

1. Miller, "Sydney Ringer: Physiological Saline, Calcium and the Contraction of the Heart."
2. McCraty and Childre, "Coherence: Bridging Personal, Social, and Global Health," 19–21.
3. *Rosch, "Job Stress: America's Leading Adult Health Problem"; *Mohd, "Life Event, Stress and Illness," 9–18.
4. Mercogliano and Debus, "The Neuroscience of the Heart," 5; McCraty, Atkinson, and Tomasino, *Science of the Heart,* 4.
5. McCraty, Atkinson, and Tomasino, *Science of the Heart,* 6–65.

Chapter 3. Building Awareness and Appreciation

1. Mitchell, *Tao Te Ching,* 33.
2. Emmons, *Thanks! How the New Science of Gratitude Can Make You Happier,* 33.
3. Ibid., 64.

Chapter 4.
Everything Is Connected to the Flow

1. Salovey and Mayer, "Emotional Intelligence," 185–211; Goleman, *Emotional Intelligence.*
2. Goleman, *Emotional Intelligence,* xix.
3. Damasio, *Descartes' Error,* 155–58.
4. McCraty, Atkinson, and Tomasino, *Science of the Heart,* 6–7.
5. Gershon, *The Second Brain.*

Chapter 6.
Everything Is Energy

1. Ueno, et al., "Noninvasive Measurement of Pulsatile Intracranial Pressure Using Ultrasound," 66–69; Ueno, et al., "Cranial Diameter Pulsation Measured by Non-Invasive Ultrasound Decrease with Tilt," 882–85. Additional sources listed at http://www.cranialacademy.com/researchBONE.html.
2. *Leary, "How to Operate Your Brain" video and transcript.
3. Milne, *Heart of Listening,* 66–205.
4. Milne, *Bone Energetics,* CD, Track 5.

Chapter 7. Becoming Liquid Light

1. Strassman, *DMT: The Spirit Molecule,* 42.
2. Schmidt, Do, Dacey, et al. "Melanopsin-Positive Intrinsically Photosensitive Retinal Ganglion Cells: From Form to Function," 16094–101.
3. Penfield, "The Role of the Temporal Cortex in Certain Psychic Phenomena," 451–65.
4. Blackmore, *Dying to Live,* 208–17.

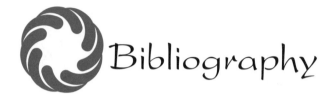 Bibliography

Amen, Daniel. *Change Your Brain, Change Your Life.* New York: Three Rivers Press, 1998.

Armour, J. Andrew, and Jeffry L. Ardell, eds. *Basic and Clinical Neuro-cardiology.* New York: Oxford University Press, 2004.

Atlee, Thomas. *Cranio-Sacral Integration: Foundation.* London: Singing Dragon, 2012.

Bartlett, Richard. *The Physics of Miracles.* New York: Atria Books, 2010.

Begley, Sharon. *Train Your Mind, Change Your Brain.* New York: Ballantine Books, 2007.

Blackmore, Susan. *Dying to Live.* New York: Prometheus Books, 1993.

Carter, Rita. *The Human Brain Book.* London: DK Adults, 2009.

Chia, Mantak. *Chi Nei Tsang.* Rochester, Vt.: Destiny Books, 2007.

———. *Tan Tien Chi Kung.* Rochester, Vt.: Destiny Books, 2004.

———. *Taoist Astral Healing.* Rochester, Vt.: Destiny Books, 2004.

Chia, Mantak, and Lee Holden. *Simple Chi Kung.* Rochester, Vt.: Destiny Books, 2011.

Chia, Mantak, and Aisha Sieburth. *Life Pulse Massage.* Rochester, Vt.: Destiny Books, 2015.

Chia, Mantak, and William U. Wei. *Sexual Reflexology.* Rochester, Vt.: Destiny Books, 2003.

Childre, D., and Martin, H. *The HeartMath Solution.* San Francisco: Harper San Francisco, 1999.

Csikszentmihalyi, Mihaly. *Flow: The Psychology of Optimum Experience.* Harper Perennial Modern Classics, 2008.

Damasio, Antonio. *Descartes' Error.* New York: Avon, 1994.

———. *The Feeling of What Happens.* New York: Harcourt, 1999.

———. *Self Comes to Mind.* New York: Vintage Books, 2010.

Deadman, Peter, and Al-Khafaji, Mazin. *A Manual of Acupuncture.* Hove, UK: Journal of Chinese Medicine Publications, 2007.

Dixon, Jana. *The Biology of Kundalini.* Lulu.com: Lulu Publishing, 2008.

Doidge, Norman. *The Brain that Changes Itself.* New York: Penguin, 2008.

Emmons, Robert. *Thanks! How the New Science of Gratitude Can Make You Happier.* New York: Houghton Mifflin, 2007.

Gershon, Michael. *The Second Brain.* New York: HarperCollins, 1998.

Goleman, Daniel. *Emotional Intelligence,* 10th anniversary ed. New York: Bantam, 2006.

Hyman, Mark. *The UltraMind Solution.* New York: Scribner, 2010.

Jealous, James. *Every Drop Knows the Tide* (CD). Apollo Beach, Fla.: Long Tide Management, 2000.

———. *Stillness 1* (CD). Apollo Beach, Fla.: Long Tide Management, 2010.

———. *Stillness 2* (CD). Apollo Beach, Fla.: Long Tide Management, 2010.

———. *The Biodynamics of Osteopathy: An Introductory Overview* (CD). Apollo Beach, Fla.: Long Tide Management, 2000.

Koch, Liz. *The Psoas Book.* Felton, Calif.: Guinea Pig Publications, 2012.

Lehrer, Jonah. *How We Decide.* New York: Houghton Mifflin Harcourt, 2009.

Lipton, Bruce. *The Biology of Belief.* Carlsbad, Calif.: Hay House Publishing, 2008.

Maciocia, Giovanni. *The Foundations of Chinese Medicine.* China: Churchill Livingstone, 2005.

———. *The Psyche in Chinese Medicine.* China: Churchill Livingstone, 2009.

McCraty, R., M. Atkinson, and D. Tomasino. *Science of the Heart.* Boulder Creek, Calif.: Institute of HeartMath, 2001.

McCraty, R., and D. Childre, "Coherence: Bridging Personal, Social, and Global Health." *Alternative Therapies* 16(4) (2010): 10–24.

Medina, John. *Brain Rules.* Seattle, Wash.: Pear Press, 2009.

Mercogliano, C., and K. Debus. "The Neuroscience of the Heart." *Journal of Family Life* 5(1) (1999). Available at http://www.ratical.org/many_worlds/JCP99.html. Last viewed August 2015.

Miller, David J. "Sydney Ringer: Physiological Saline, Calcium and the Contraction of the Heart." *Journal of Physiology* 555(Pt 3) (2004): 585–87. Available at http://www.ncbi.nlm.nih.gov/pmc/articles/PMC1664856/. Last viewed August 2015.

Milne, Hugh. *Bone Energetics* (CD). Big Sur, Calif.: Milne Institute, 2006.

———. *The Heart of Listening: A Visionary Approach to Craniosacral Work.* Berkeley, Calif.: North Atlantic Books, 1996.

Mitchell, Stephen. *Tao Te Ching.* New York, HarperCollins, 1988.

Netter, Frank H. *Atlas of Human Anatomy.* 5th ed. Philadelphia: Saunders, 2010.

Parker, Steve, and Robert Winston. *The Human Body Book.* London: DK Adults, 2007.

Paxinos, George, ed. *The Human Nervous System.* San Diego, Calif.: Academic Press, 1990.

Pearsall, Paul. *The Heart's Code.* New York: Broadway Books, 1998.

Penfield, Wilder. "The Role of the Temporal Cortex in Certain Psychical Phenomena." *Journal of Mental Science* 101(424) (1955): 451–65. Available at http://bjp.rcpsych.org/content/101/424/451. Last viewed August 2015.

Rock, David. *Your Brain at Work.* New York: Harper Collins e-books, 2009.

Salovey, P., and J. D. Mayer. "Emotional Intelligence." *Imagination, Cognition, and Personality* 9 (1990): 185–211. Available at http://ei.yale.edu/wp-content/uploads/2014/06/pub153_SaloveyMayerICP1990_OCR.pdf. Last viewed August 2015.

Schmidt, T. M., M. T. H. Do, D. Dacey, et al. "Melanopsin-Positive Intrinsically Photosensitive Retinal Ganglion Cells: From Form to Function." *Journal of Neuroscience* 31(45) (2011): 16094–101. Available at http://www.ncbi.nlm.nih.gov/pmc/articles/PMC3267581/. Last viewed August 2015.

Sherwood, Ben. *The Survivors Club.* New York: Grand Central Publishing, 2010.

Siegel, Daniel J. *The Mindful Brain.* New York & Boston: W. W. Norton & Company, 2007.

———. *The Mindful Therapist*. New York: W.W. Norton & Company, 2010.

———. *MindSight*. New York: Bantam, 2010.

Sills Franklyn. *Foundations in Craniosacral Biodynamics*. Vol. 1. Berkeley, Calif.: North Atlantic Books, 2011.

Strassman, Rick. *DMT: The Spirit Molecule: A Doctor's Revolutionary Research into the Biology of Near-Death and Mystical Experiences*. Rochester, Vt.: Park Street Press, 2000.

Ueno, T., R. E. Ballard, B. R. Macias, et al. "Cranial Diameter Pulsation Measured by Non-Invasive Ultrasound Decrease with Tilt." *Aviation, Space and Environmental Medicine* 74(8) (2003): 882–85. Available at http://www.researchgate.net/publication/10608543_Cranial_diameter _pulsations_measured_by_non-invasive_ultrasound_decrease_with _tilt. Last viewed August 2015.

Ueno, T., R. E. Ballard, L. M. Shuer, et al. "Noninvasive Measurement of Pulsatile Intracranial Pressure Using Ultrasound." *Acta Neurochirurgica* 71 (suppl.) (1998): 66–69. Available at http://link.springer.com /chapter/10.1007/978-3-7091-6475-4_21. Last viewed August 2015.

Venes, Don. *Taber's Cyclopedic Medical Dictionary*. Philadelphia: F. A. Davis Company, 2009.

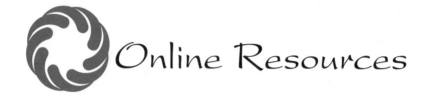 Online Resources

Barren, Jon. "The Endocrine System: Hypothalamus, Pituitary, and Pineal Glands." (2010). Available at http://jonbarron.org/article/endocrine-system-hypothalamus-pituitary-pineal-glands. Last viewed August 2015.

Bowen, R. "The Pineal Gland and Melatonin." (2003). Available at http://www.vivo.colostate.edu/hbooks/pathphys/endocrine/otherendo/pineal.html. Last viewed July 2015.

Cook, Andrew. "The SBS Revisited: The Mechanics of Cranial Motion." (2004). Available at http://www.academia.edu/6066991/The_mechanics_of_cranial_motion_the_sphenobasilar_synchondrosis_SBS_revisited. Last viewed July 2015.

Glassey, Don. "Life Energy and Healing." (2011). Available at http://www.ofspirit.com/donglassey1.htm. Last viewed July 2015.

———. "Why Yoga Works." (2010). Available at http://www.ofspirit.com/donglassey4.htm. Last viewed July 2015.

Institute of HeartMath. "Science of The Heart: Exploring the Role of the Heart in Human Performance: An Overview of Research Conducted by the Institute of HeartMath." (2001). Available at https://www.heartmath.org/resources/downloads/science-of-the-heart/. Last viewed July 2015.

Lan, Fengli. "Understanding Shen in Classical Chinese Texts." (n.d.) Available at http://shenjiva.com/Understanding-SHEN-in-Classical-Chinese-Texts11.pdf. Last viewed August 2015.

LearnersDictionary.com. "Learner's definition of FLOW." Available at http://www.learnersdictionary.com/definition/flow. Last viewed August 2015.

Leary, Timothy. "How to Operate Your Brain." (1993). Video available at http://www.openculture.com/2012/11/how_to_operate_your

_brain_a_user_manual_by_timothy_leary_.html. Transcript available at http://visions.cz/audiovisual-performance/Timothy-Leary-How-to-operate-your-brain. Last viewed August 2015.

Levi, Renee. "The Sentient Heart: Messages for Life." (2001). Available at http://www.resonanceproject.org/concept3.cfm?pt=2. Last viewed July 2015.

Maciocia, Giovanni. "Mirror Neurons: The Arena of Shen and Hun." (2012). Available at http://maciociaonline.blogspot.com/2012/02 /mirror-neurons-arena-of-shen-and-hun.html. Last viewed July 2015.

McCraty, Rollin. "The Energetic Heart." (2003). Available at https:// www.heartmath.org/gci/resources/downloads/the-energetic-heart-gci-edition/. Last viewed July 2015.

———. "The Scientific Role of the Heart in Learning and Performance." (2003). Available at https://www.heartmath.org/assets/uploads/2015/01 /scientific-role-of-the-heart.pdf. Last viewed July 2015.

McCraty, R., M. Atkinson, D. Tomasino, et al. "The electricity of touch: Detection and Measurement of Cardiac Energy Exchange between People." (1998). Available at https://www.heartmath.org/research/research-library/energetics/electricity-of-touch/. Last viewed July 2015.

Merriam-Webster.com. "Full Definition of Flow." Available at http://www .merriam-webster.com/dictionary/flow. Last viewed August 2015.

Miller, Iona. "Soma Pinoline: Blinded by the Light." (2006). Available at http://ionamiller.weebly.com/pineal-dmt.html. Last viewed July 2015.

Miller, Julie Ann. "Eye to (Third) Eye." (1985). Available at http://www .highbeam.com/doc/1G1-4016492.html. Last viewed July 2015.

Mohd, Razali Salleh. "Life Event, Stress and Illness." (2008). Available at http://www.ncbi.nlm.nih.gov/pmc/articles/PMC3341916/. Last viewed August 2015.

Morgan, Steven. "Rethinking the Potential of the Brain in Major Psychiatric Disorders." (2008). Available at http://www.mindfreedom.org/kb /diagnostics/rethinking-the-brain. Last viewed July 2015.

Porges, Stephen. "The Polyvagal Perspective." (2007). Available at http:// stephenporges.com/images/polyvagal_perspective.pdf. Last viewed July 2015.

———. "Somatic Perspectives on Psychotherapy." (2011). Available at http://www.stephenporges.com/images/somatic%20perspectives%20 porges.pdf. Last viewed August 2015.

Roney-Dougal, Serena. "Walking Between the Worlds: Links between Psi, Psychedelics, Shamanism and Psychosis. An Overview of the Literature." (2012). Available at http://www.psi-researchcentre.co.uk /article_1.html. Last viewed July 2015.

Rosch, Paul J. "Job Stress: America's Leading Adult Health Problem." (1991). Available at http://www.stress.org/americas-1-health-problem/. Last viewed August 2015.

Unq, C. Y. and Molteno, A. C. "An enigmatic eye: the histology of the tuatara pineal complex." (2004). Available at http://www.ncbi.nlm.nih .gov/pubmed/15633271. Last viewed July 2015.

Whedon, James M., DC. "Cerebrospinal Fluid Stasis and Its Clinical Significance." (2009). Available at http://www.ncbi.nlm.nih.gov /pubmed/19472865. Last viewed July 2015.

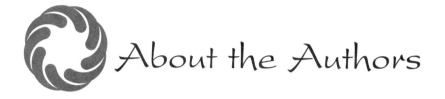

About the Authors

MANTAK CHIA

Mantak Chia has been studying the Taoist approach to life since childhood. His mastery of this ancient knowledge, enhanced by his study of other disciplines, has resulted in the development of the Universal Healing Tao system, which is now being taught throughout the world.

Mantak Chia was born in Thailand to Chinese parents in 1944. When he was six years old, he learned from Buddhist monks how to sit and "still the mind." While in grammar school he learned traditional Thai boxing, and he soon went on to acquire considerable skill in aikido, yoga, and Tai Chi. His studies of the Taoist way of life began in earnest when he was a student in Hong Kong, ultimately leading to his mastery of a wide variety of esoteric disciplines, with the guidance of several masters, including Master I Yun, Master Meugi, Master Cheng Yao Lun, and Master Pan Yu. To better understand the mechanisms behind healing energy, he also studied Western anatomy and medical sciences.

Master Chia has taught his system of healing and energizing practices to tens of thousands of students and trained more than two thousand instructors and practitioners throughout the world. He has established centers for Taoist study and training in many countries around the globe. In June of 1990, he was honored by the International Congress of Chinese Medicine and Qi Gong (Chi Kung), which named him the Qi Gong Master of the Year.

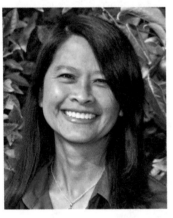

JOYCE THOM

As founder and director of ThePATH. us, Joyce is passionate about sharing her thirty plus years of experience in meditation, energy cultivation, and the healing arts. She teaches seminars around the world in Craniosacral Work, Chi Kung, consciousness studies, energy skills, and traditional Asian therapies.

Joyce began studying meditation, acupressure, and Qi cultivation as a student of martial arts in 1979. Since 1986, she has focused on the healing aspects of these ancient Eastern practices. She holds a Masters of Medical Qi Gong from the International Institute of Medical Qi Gong and advanced certification in Traditional Asian Therapies from the Acupressure Institute, where she was on the faculty for nine years. Joyce has been fascinated with the Taoist approach to life since her youth and began studying Master Chia's Universal Healing Tao system in 2002.

Trained in several modern Western healing arts, Joyce integrates the best of both worlds into her sessions and workshops. She began her craniosacral journey at the Heartwood and Upledger Institutes and deepened her practice with biodynamic and Visionary CranioSacral Work at the Milne Institute, where she has been an instructor since 2007. Her clear and compassionate style invites and inspires people to fulfill more and more of their potential.

Joyce has a B.A. from Yale and an M.P.A. in public and international affairs from Princeton. Prior to focusing on her private practice and teaching, Joyce was a senior executive in general management, strategy, and marketing at leading Silicon Valley companies. In the 1990s, she cofounded and was CEO of a technology company that developed and patented innovations in the field of data infrastructure. With her years of experience in high-pressure environments, Joyce emphasizes the importance of staying balanced, centered, and fluid so we can continue to be effective, creative, and radiantly healthy throughout our lives. For more information, visit **www.ThePATH.us**.

The Universal Healing Tao System and Training Center

THE UNIVERSAL HEALING TAO SYSTEM

The ultimate goal of Taoist practice is to transcend physical boundaries through the development of the soul and the spirit within the human. That is also the guiding principle behind the Universal Healing Tao, a practical system of self-development that enables individuals to complete the harmonious evolution of their physical, mental, and spiritual bodies. Through a series of ancient Chinese meditative and internal energy exercises, the practitioner learns to increase physical energy, release tension, improve health, practice self-defense, and gain the ability to heal him- or herself and others. In the process of creating a solid foundation of health and well-being in the physical body, the practitioner also creates the basis for developing his or her spiritual potential by learning to tap in to the natural energies of the sun, moon, earth, stars, and other environmental forces.

The Universal Healing Tao practices are derived from ancient techniques rooted in the processes of nature. They have been gathered and integrated into a coherent, accessible system for well-being that works directly with the life force, or chi, that flows through the meridian system of the body.

Master Chia has spent years developing and perfecting techniques for teaching these traditional practices to students around the world through ongoing classes, workshops, private instruction, and healing sessions, as well as books and video and audio products. Further information can be obtained at www.universal-tao.com.

THE UNIVERSAL HEALING TAO TRAINING CENTER

The Tao Garden Resort and Training Center in northern Thailand is the home of Master Chia and serves as the worldwide headquarters for Universal Healing Tao activities. This integrated wellness, holistic health, and training center is situated on eighty acres surrounded by the beautiful Himalayan foothills near the historic walled city of Chiang Mai. The serene setting includes flower and herb gardens ideal for meditation, open-air pavilions for practicing Chi Kung, and a health and fitness spa.

The center offers classes year round, as well as summer and winter retreats. It can accommodate two hundred students, and group leasing can be arranged. For information on courses, books, products, and other resources, see below.

RESOURCES

Universal Healing Tao Center
274 Moo 7, Laung Nua, Doi Saket, Chiang Mai, 50220, Thailand
Tel: (66)(53) 921-200
E-mail: universaltao@universal-tao.com
Web site: www.universal-tao.com

For information on retreats and the health spa, contact:
Tao Garden Health Spa & Resort
E-mail: reservations@tao-garden.com
Web site: www.tao-garden.com

Good Chi • Good Heart • Good Intention

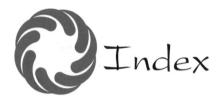# Index

Page numbers in *italics* indicate illustrations and photographs.

American Institute of Stress, 32

asculta (listening), 100

atrial natriuretic factor (ANF), 91

awareness and appreciation
  Appreciating the Pumps, 76–77, *76*
  Connecting the Pumps, 72–73, *72, 73*
  Connecting to the Core Link, 68–70, *69, 70*
  and Flow, signs of improvement in, 74
  Following the Breath, 64–66, *66*
  health benefits of, 74–75, *75*
  Inner Smile, 76–77, *76*

balance, and tracking the Flow, *17,* 18

Beauchene skull, 148, *149*

belly
  Chi Nei Tsang Self-Message, 124–26, *125*
  Empty Force Breathing, 122–23, *123*

bladder. *See* urinary bladder

blood flow, 28, *29,* 35–36, *35*

blood pressure, 28, 36

body
  and Flow, 11–16
  benefits of Craniosacral Work, 16–19

wisdom, 19–20

bone of light consciousness, 159, *160, 161*

bones
  Bone Breathing, 169–70
  effect on mood and memory, 147
  electrical charge in, 144–45
  mobility and motility, 147–50, *149, 150*
  sensing energy in, 145–46
  Shaking the Bones, 146
  wisdom of, 143–44, *143, 144*
  See also cranium

brain
  orbitofrontal areas, 87
  psoas muscle and, 112, *112*
  reptilian, 112, *112,* 144
  temporal lobes, 207
  three brains, 89–96
  See also cranium; gut brain; head brain; heart brain

breathing
  Abdominal or Natural Breathing, 28–29, *29*
  Breathing into the Heart, 39–40, *40*
  Breath of Life, 19–20, 27–28, 37–38, *37,* 46, 222, *222,* 226

Following the Breath, 64–66, *66*
  reverse, 29–30, *30*
  shallow, 20
  Spinal Cord Breathing, 58–59, *59, 205–7*
  Taoist breathing methods, 26–30

cardiac pump, *25,* 30–34, *31, 33*
cardiac and respiratory pumps, 35–40, *35, 37, 39, 40*
Celestial Pillar, 22–24, *22*
central nervous system, 43–44, *43*
cerebrospinal fluid (CSF)
  cardiac and respiratory pumps and, 40, 41, *41*
  in craniosacral system, 44–47, *45*
  enlightenment experiences and, 206
  Flow and, 15
  mental-emotional balance and, 46
  sacral pump and, 41
  sphenoid and sacrum and, 156, *157*
Chi Kung, 1–3, 71
  Chi Kung Breathing, 37–38, *37*
  and Craniosacral Work, 205–7
  and Crystal Palace activation, 202, *203,* 204–5
  Inner Smile, 76–77, *76*
  regulating emotions and emotional intelligence, 82, 86
chi (life-force energy), 13, 24
ching (essence), 24
Chuang Tzu, 223, *223*
circadian rhythms, 14, 192, 194, 200, 202
coccyx, described, 41, *42*
cognitive psychology, 86

communication
  in body, and cerebrospinal fluid (CSF), 45–46
  and Flow between body structures, 12
connection
  in body, and cerebrospinal fluid (CSF), 45–46
  Connecting to the Core Link, 68–71, *69, 70*
  Connecting the Pumps, 72–73, *72, 73*
  and Flow between body structures, 11–12
  Microcosmic Orbit, 175–78, *176*
  Riding the Horse, 172–73, *173*
  Swimming Dragon, 173–75, *175*
connective tissue and mediastinum, 38–39, *39*
consciousness
  bone of light consciousness, 159–61, *160,* 172
  Flow (waves and tides) and, 208–14
  heart's electromagnetic field and, 206
  melatonin and, 198
  perceptions and, 87–88
  personal star and, 220
  physical Flow and, 16
  Yin and Yang Breathing, 225–27, *225*
  See also spiritual experiences
Core Link, 47
  activating, 58–63, *59, 60, 61, 62*
  Connecting to the Core Link, 68–71, *69, 70*
  gut brain, or lower tan tien and, 95
Cosmic Flow
  Becoming the Cosmic Flow, 237–39, *238*

cosmic flows of energy, 14

Crane, 60, *61*

exercises, other, for activating, 63

Spinal Cord Breathing, 58–59, *59*, 205–7

Turtle, 61, *61*

Wagging the Dragon's Tail, 62, *62*

cranial osteopathy, 20

cranial pump, *25*, 41, *41*

Activating the Cranial Pump, 56–57, *57*

Bending the Neck, 54, *54*

opening, 53–57

Rocking the Neck, 54, *54*

Rolling the Neck, 56, *56*

Rotating the Neck, 55, *55*

Cranial Wave, 20, 101

Connecting to the Core Link, 68–71, *69, 70*

cranial motility, 152

Craniosacral Work, 208–9, *208*, 211

cranium to sacrum, 68

Craniosacral Work, 1–3

bones of the cranium, 148, *149*, 150–58

Breath of Life, 19–20

and Chi Kung, 205–7, 239

following the flow, 101–2

four waves and tides, 208–11, *208–11*

listening with the heart, 99–100

Push Hands exercises, 104–10, *106, 107, 109, 110*

tracking the Flow, 16–19, *17, 18*

unwinding the knots, 102–4, *103*

cranium, 41, *41*

Activating the Cranial Pump, 56–57, *57*

Cranial Bone Sensing, 170–72

Feeling Cranial Motility, 152

flexion and extension of, 150–52, *151*

foramun magnum, 156, *156*

frontal bone, 164, *165*

mandible, 167–68, *168*

maxillae, 166, *167*

mobility and motility of bones in, 148, *149*, 150

occiput, 24, 41, *41*, 43, *43*, 68, 69, 71, 148, *164*

parietals, 165, *165*

sphenobasilar joint (SBJ), 154, *154, 155*, 156

sphenoid, 152–54, *153, 154, 155*, 156, *157*

temporals, 166, *166*

See also brain; Crystal Palace; eyes; spine; tan tiens

Crystal Palace

activating, 201–5

hydration and, 205

hypothalamus, pineal, and pituitary glands, 201–5, *201, 203*

relationship with light, 201–2

Dark Matter, as energy source, 143

depression, 15, 74–75

diaphragm, 26–27, 39

DMT, the Spirit Molecule, 198

dura mater

Core Link and, 58–63

craniosacral system, 43–44, *43*

eating and circadian rhythms, 14
Einstein, Albert, 142
electrocardiogram (ECG), 12
electroencephalogram (EEG), 12
electromagnetic field
    and Flow, 12
    and heart, 12, 32–33, *33,* 90, 200, 239
    North Star, 199
    Spinal Cord Breathing, 58–59, *59,*
        205–7
    Spiraling, 204
emotional intelligence, 84–88, *85, 88*
Emotional Intelligence (Goleman), 85–86
emotions
    accessing Flow of, 81–84
    challenging, gifts of, 84
    Craniosacral Work and, 99–104
    Empty Force Breathing, 122–23, *123*
    five elements and, 83–84, *83,* 96,
        96, 97
    healing, physical, and effects, 88
    heart brain and, 89–92, *90, 92*
    hypothalamus/pituitary relationship,
        192–95, *193*
    introduction to Flow of, 15, 79–80
    perceptions and, 86–88, *88*
    psoas muscle, relaxing, 113–14
    Yin Breathing, 115–16
endocrine system, 158, *159*
    biological functions of, 191–192
    hypothalamus/pituitary relationship,
        192–95, *193*
    pineal gland, 195–200, *196, 197,*
        198, 200, 201, 201
energy
    cranial flexion and extension,
        150–59

Dark Matter, 143
    and Flow, 13, 172–78
    increasing, 28, *29*
    mandible and, 167–68
    meridians, 178–90
    sacrum and, 168–69, *169*
    stuck in cranium, 164
    wisdom in our bones, 143–50
enlightenment
    pineal gland, 176, 196–97, 206
    pituitary gland, 206
    sacrum, 168
enteric nervous system, 93–94
exercises
    Abdominal or Natural Breathing,
        28–29, *29*
    Activating the Cranial Pump,
        56–57, *57*
    Appreciating the Pumps, 76–77, *76*
    Awakening the Sacral Pump, 50–51,
        51
    Becoming the Cosmic Flow, 237–
        39, *238*
    Bending the Neck, 54, *54*
    Bone Breathing, 169–70
    Breathing into the Heart, 39–40, *40*
    Brushing the Yin and Yang
        Meridians, 180–82, *181*
    Chi Kung Breath of Life, 37–38, *37*
    Combining the Three Tan Tiens,
        215–16, *216*
    Connecting to the Core Link,
        68–71, *69, 70*
    Connecting the Pumps, 72–73, *72, 73*
    Crane, 60, *61*
    Cranial Bone Sensing, 170–72
    Empty Force Breathing, 122–23, *123*

Expanding to the Six Directions, 216–22, *217–22*

Feeling Cranial Motility, 152

Filling the Sacral Pump, 52–53, *52*

Fire Dragon, 174–75

Flowing between Empty and Full, 228–29, *228*

Following the Breath, 64–66, *66*

Following the Clock, 161–62

Heart's Sound—Fire Element, The, 135–36, *136*

Kidneys' Sound—Water Element, The, 132–33, *132*

Laughter Chi Kung, 128–30, *129*

Listening to the Heart Flow, 66–67, *67*

Listening with the Heart to the Psoas Muscle, 116–18, *117*

Liver's Sound—Wood Element, The, 133–35, *134*

Lungs' Sound—Metal Element, The, 130–32, *131*

Microcosmic Orbit, 175–78, *176*

Opening the Hips, 48, *49*

Opening the Waist, 48, *48*

Psoas Muscle Release, 118–21, *119, 120*

Pull the Bow and Shoot the Arrow, 234–36, *235*

Push Hands exercises, 104–10, *106, 107, 109, 110*, 231–32, *231*

Reverse Breathing, 29–30, *30*

Riding the Horse, 172–73, *173*

Rocking the Neck, 54, *54*

Rolling the Neck, 56, *56*

Rotating the Neck, 55, *55*

Rotating the Sacrum, 49–50, *50*

Shaking the Bones, 146

Spinal Cord Breathing, 58–59, *59, 205–7*

Spleen's Sound—Earth Element, The, 136–38, *137*

Sustaining the Flow, 77–78, *78*

Swimming Dragon, 173–75, *175*

Tapping the Heart, 34

Tracing the Meridian Flow, 182–90, *183–89*

Triple Warmer's Sound, The, 138–39, *138*

Turtle, 61, *61*

Wagging the Dragon's Tail, 62, *62*

Warm-Ups for the World Link Meditation, 214–15

Yin and Yang Breathing, 225–27, *225*

Yin Breathing, 115–16

exhalation

balancing heart and lungs, 36–37

extension of cranial bones during, 150–52, *151*

respiratory pump and, 27, *27*

sphenobasilar joint (SBJ) and, 154, *155*

See also breathing

eyes

bone of light consciousness, 159, *160*, 161

Crystal Palace and, *201*, 201–2

Following the Clock, 161–62

gazing, 161

fascia, and Craniosacral Work, 104

Fenwick, Peter, 207

fight-or-flight reaction

heart rate, effect on, 31, *31*

hypothalamus and, 192–94, *193*
psoas muscle and, 112
five elements
and emotions, 83–84, *83*
and organs of the body, 96, *96, 97*
flexibility
Chi Nei Tsang self-massage, 126
psoas muscle and, 111–13, *111, 113*
Spinal Cord Breathing, 58–59, *59, 205–7*
temporal bones and, 166, *166*
Flow
benefits of, 11–16
Combining the Three Tan Tiens, 215, *216*
Cranial Wave, 68
Fire Dragon, 174–75, *175*
Flowing between Empty and Full, 228–29, *228*
Following the Breath, 64–66, *66*
four characteristics of, 16–19, *17, 18*
introduction to, 2–5
levers, three, for accessing, 97–98
liquid light, becoming, *221*
Listening to the Heart Flow, 66–67, *67*
Microcosmic Orbit, 175–78, *176*
natural rhythms and, 13–14, *13*
physical, and signs of improvement, 74
physical benefits of, 11–13
Riding the Horse, 174–75, *175*
Sustaining the Flow, 77–78, *78*
Swimming Dragon, 173–74, *174*
See also meridians
Fluid Tide, 20, 176, 209, *209*, 215, *216*, 226

following the Flow
in Craniosacral Work, 101–2, *102*
Push Hands: Following, 107–8, *107*
foramun magnum, 156, *156*
frontal bone of cranium, 164, *165*

gall bladder, 179–81, *180, 181*, 188, *188*
gates of the spine (Celestial Pillar), 22, 23–24, *23*. *See also* tan tiens
gazing, 161. *See also* eyes
Gershon, Michael, 93–94
Goleman, Daniel, 84, 85–86
gratitude, health benefits of, 74–75, *75*
gut brain, 93–95, *93*

head brain, 89, *89, 94–95*. *See also* brain; heart brain; gut brain
health
abdominal breathing and, 28, *29*
benefits of appreciation, 74–75, 175
heart
asculta (listening), 100
awakening, 34
Breathing into the Heart, 39–40, *40*
cardiac pump, 30–34, *31, 33*
electromagnetic field of, 32–33, *33*
Listening to the Heart Flow, 66–67, *67*
and lungs, 35–40, *39, 40*
mediastinum and, 38–39, *39*
meridian, 179–85, *180, 181, 185*
and pineal gland, 200
in Upanishads, 33–34
heart brain, 89–93, *90, 92*
HeartMath Institute, 32–33, 91
HeartMind concept, 86
Heart of Listening (Milne), 162

heart rate, slowing with abdominal
breathing, 28
Heart's Sound—Fire Element, The,
135–36, *136*
hips
Opening the Hips, 48, *49*
psoas muscle and, 121
hormones
hypothalamus/pituitary relationship,
192–95, *193*
pituitary gland, 194–95
Hui Yin (perineum), 29, *30*
hypothalamus gland
Crystal Palace, 201, *201*
and pituitary, 192–95, *193*, 201, *201*
suprachiasmatic nucleus (SCN), 202

immune system
atrial natriuretic factor (ANF), 91
cerebrospinal fluid (CSF) and, 63
gratitude and, 75
reverse breathing and, 29–30, *30*
inhalation
balancing heart and lungs, 36–37
flexion of cranial bones during,
150–52, *151*
and laughter, benefits of, 128
and respiratory pump, 27, *27*
sphenobasilar joint (SBJ), 154, *155*
See also breathing
Inner Smile, 21, 76–78, *76, 78*

Jade Pillow Pass (Yu Zhen Guan or
upper gate), 23, *24*
Jia Jin Guan (Squeeze the Spine Pass or
middle gate), 23, *24*
joining the Flow, 212–14, *213*

Karsenty, Gerard, 147
kidneys
elements and emotions, 96–97, *97*
lotus meditation, for refreshing,
114–15, *115*
meridian, 179–81, *180, 181*, 186,
186
Refreshing Lotus Meditation, 114–
15, *115*
Reverse Breathing, 29–30, *30*
Kidney's Sound—Water Element, The
132–33, *132*
knots, unwinding
in Craniosacral Work, 102–4
Push Hands: Noticing the Direction
of Movement, 108–9, *109*

Lao Tzu, 64, 233
large intestine, 179–83, *180, 181, 183*
Laughter Chi Kung, 128–30, *129*
Leary, Timothy, 161
letting go
Pull the Bow and Shoot the Arrow,
234–36, *235*
light
and glands in cranium, 201
and pineal gland, 198
liquid light, 207, 210
listening
in Craniosacral Work, 99–100
Push Hands: Listening, 105–6, *106*
Push Hands: Moving into Stillness,
231–32, *231*
Push Hands: Unwinding, 109–10,
109
Liver meridian, 179–81, *180, 181*,
188, *188*

Liver's Sound—Wood Element, The, 133–35, *134*

Long Tide, 20, 210, *210,* 216–22, *217–22,* 226

Long Wave, 20, 211, *211,* 227

lower gate (Wei Lu Guan or Tailbone Pass), 23, *23*

lower tan tien and abdominal breathing, *27,* 28, *29*

lungs
Chi Kung Breathing, 37–38, *37*
and heart, 35–40, *39, 40*
increasing capacity, with reverse breathing, 29–30, *30*
meridian flow, 179–80, *181*, 183, *183,* 189, *189*

Lung's Sound—Metal Element, The, 130–32, *131*

magnetic fields and pineal gland, 199–200, *200*

magnitude, and tracking the Flow, *17,* 18

Maman, Fabien, 199

massage
Chi Nei Tsang Self-Massage, 123–26, *125*

Mayer, John, 84

mediastenum, 38–39, *39*

meditation
Crystal Palace, 201
DMT produced by, 198
and emotional intelligence, 85
Inner Smile, 76–77, *76*
Lotus Meditation, 114–15, *115*
Six Healing Sounds, 130–39

Warm-Ups for the World Link Meditation, 214–15

World Link Mediation, 214–23

medulla oblongata, 156, 164

melatonin, 195, 198, *198,* 202, 204, 207

mental health
and Flow, 15–16, 126–30
six sounds for balance, 130–39

meridians
Brushing the Yin and Yang Meridians, 180–82, *181*
Flow, described, 179
meridian body clock, 179, *179, 180*
Tracing the Meridian Flow, 182–90, *183–89*

Microcosmic Orbit, 24, 176–78, *176*

middle gate (Jia Jin Guan or Squeeze the Spine Pass), *23,* 24

Milne, Hugh, 162

movement, toward ease and toward discomfort, 101–2

"muscle of the soul" (psoas muscle), 11–14

neck
cranial pump, opening, 53–57
mandible and, 167–68
tension in, 53, *53,* 168

negative emotions
and mental Flow, 81–84, *82, 83, 84*
six sounds for balance, 130–39

Neppe, Vernon, 207

nervous system
sensory, and Flow, 12

neurotransmitters
endocrine system and, 192

and gut brain, 94
and heart brain, 90
No Mind, 232–33
North Star, 199, 227, *227*

occipital bone of cranium
  and cerebrospinal fluid, 41, *41*
  energetics of, 163–64, *164*
  in harmony with sacrum, 69, *69*
  and sphenoid, 154, *155*
optic system
  Crystal Palace, 201–5, *201, 203*
  and glands in cranium, 193, *193*
  sphenoid and, *160,* 161
organs of the body
  and five elements and emotions, 96,
    96, 97
  gaze and effect on healing, 161
  meridians, 178–95, *179, 180, 181*
  Six Healing Sounds for Mental
    Balance, 130–39
Original Spirit, 33–34
osteopathy, cranial, 20
oxytocin, 89

parasympathetic nervous system, 31
  sacral nerves and, 51
Penfield, Wilder, 207
perception, formed by sensing, thinking,
  and feeling, 86–88, *88*
pericardium, 179–81, *180, 181,* 187, *187*
pineal gland, 195–200, *196, 197, 198,
  200*
pituitary gland
  and Crystal Palace, 201, *201*
  hormones, 194–95
  and sphenoid, 158, *158*

psoas muscle
  described, 111–13, *111, 112, 113*
  Listening with the Heart to the
    Psoas Muscle, 116–18, *117*
  Psoas Muscle Release, 118–21, *119,
    120*
pumps, four major
  cardiac and respiratory pumps,
    35–40, *35, 37, 39, 40*
  cardiac pump, 30–34, *31, 33*
  cranial pump, 41, *41*
  respiratory pump, 26–30, *27, 29, 30*
  sacral pump, 41, *42*
  See also gates of the spine; tan tiens
pulses
  North Star, 199
  reading, in Asian medicine, 13
  Yin and Yang Breathing, 225–27,
    225, 227
Push Hands exercises, 104–10, *106,
  107, 109, 110*

quality, and tracking the Flow, *17,* 18

relationship management, 84–85
relaxation, and tracking the Flow, 19
resilience and Flow, 12
resonance (rhythm entrainment), 199
respiratory pump, *25,* 26–30, *27, 29,
  30*

sacral nerves, 51–52
sacral pump, *25,* 41, *42,* 47–50
  Awakening the Sacral Pump, 50–51,
    50, 51
  Filling the Sacral Pump, 52–53, *52*
  sacral nerves and, 51–52

sacrum
  in abdominal/natural breathing, 28, 29
  described, 41, *42*
  energetics of, 168–69, *169*
  in harmony with occiput, 69, *69*
  in reverse breathing, 29–30, *30*
  Rotating the Sacrum, 49–50, *50*
  sacral nerves and, 51
  and sphenoid, 156, *157*
Saint Benedict, 100
Salovey, Peter, 84
sciatic nerve, 52
self-awareness, 84
self-healing in Craniosacral Work, 11
self-management, 84–85
sella turcica, 158
sensing
  energy in bones, 145–46
  as part of perceptions, 86–88, *88*
serotonin and other neurochemicals, 195–96
shen (spirit) and Celestial Pillar, 24
sinoatrial node (SA node), 30–31, *31*, 34
Six Healing Sounds for Mental Balance, 130–39
skull. *See* cranium
sleep and circadian rhythms, 14
small intestine, 179–85, *180, 181, 185*
social awareness, 84–85
sound
  and electromagnetic field, 199
  Six Healing Sounds for Mental Balance, 130–39, *131–38*
  vibration and healing, 199
Source, 33–34

sphenoid
  bone of light consciousness, 159, *160,* 161
  energetics of, 163
  master bone of cranium, 152–54, *153, 154, 155,* 156
  and pituitary gland, 158, *158*
spine
  as Celestial Pillar, 22–24, *22*
  and dura mater, 43–44, *43*
  psoas muscle and, 111–14
  Spinal Cord Breathing, 58–59, *59, 205–7*
  See also tan tiens
spirit molecules, 198, *198*
spiritual experiences
  Expanding to the Six Directions, 216–22, *217–22*
  natural, 205–7
  No Mind, 232–33
  Pull the Bow and Shoot the Arrow, 234–36, *235, 236*
  states of consciousness and, 208–14
  wisdom in our bones and, 143–50
  World Link meditation, 214–22
spleen, 179–84, *180, 181, 184*
Spleen's Sound—Earth Element, The, 136–38, *137*
Squeeze the Spine Pass (Jia Jin Guan or middle gate), *23,* 24
Still, Andrew Taylor, 46
stomach, 179–84, *180, 181, 184*
Strassman, Rick, 198
stress, 32, 53, 94–95, 111–13, *111, 112, 113*
Sutherland, William Garner, 20, 148

sympathetic nervous system
  forming perceptions, 86–87, *87*
  heart rate and, 31
Tai Chi
  activating the Core Link, 63, 71
  concepts of Flow, 104–6, *106*
  for observing tension and challenging
    emotions, 82
  psoas muscle exercises, 121–22
  Push Hands exercises, 104–10, *106,*
    107, 109, 110
Tailbone Pass (Wei Lu Guan or lower
  gate), 23, *22, 23*
tan tiens
  cardiac and respiratory pumps,
    35–40, *35, 37, 39, 40*
  cardiac pump, 30–34, *31, 33*
  Combining the Three Tan Tiens,
    215, *216*
  cranial pump, 41, *41*
  liquid light ambrosia and, 207
  lower gate, 23, *23, 27,* 28
  middle gate, *23,* 24
  respiratory pump, 26–30, *27, 29,*
    30
  sacral pump, 41, *42*
  three brains and, 89–95, *89*
  three pumps or tan tiens, *25*
  upper gate, *23,* 24
Tan Tien Chi Kung, and activating the
  Core Link, 63
Tao Garden, 1, 263
Taoism
  balanced approach of, 212–14
  breathing methods of, 26–30
  and chi or life-force energy, 13, 20
  wisdom of Flow and, 21–24, *22*

tempo, and tracking the Flow, 16, *17*
third eye, 197
thoughts and perceptions, 86–88, *88*
Thuban, pulse of, 226, *227*
toxins, eliminating, 28, 36–37, 124
Triple Warmer meridian, 179–81, *180,*
  181, 187, *187*
Triple Warmer's Sound, The, 138–39,
  138
tryptophan, 205
Turtle, 61, *61*

Universal Healing Tao practices, 1, 26,
  46, 63, 80, 85
University of Connecticut, 74–75
unwinding knots
  Craniosacral Work, 102–4, *103*
  Tai Chi "Push Hands" exercises,
    104–10, *106, 107, 109, 110*
upper gate (Yu Zhen Guan or Jade
  Pillow Pass), *23,* 24
urinary bladder, 52, 179–81, *180, 181,*
  186, *186*

Vega, pulse of, 226, *227*
Visionary Craniosacral Work, 211

waist, and exercise to open, 48, *48*
Wei Lu Guan (lower gate or Tailbone
  Pass), 23, *22, 23*
wisdom traditions, 19–20, 127–28
World Link meditation, 214–22
Wu Wei, 224

Yu Zhen Guan (Jade Pillow Pass or
  upper gate), *23,* 24